Clinical Reflexology

For Churchill Livingstone

Publishing Manager, Health Professions: Inta Ozols
Project Manager: Jane Dingwall
Design Direction: Judith Wright

Clinical Reflexology
A Guide for Health Professionals

Edited by

Peter A Mackereth MA RGN CertEd DipNurs DipReflex
MCAR AdvReflex (Level3)
Lecturer and Practitioner in Complementary Therapies, Christie Hospital and
University of Salford, Manchester, UK

Denise Tiran MSc RGN RM ADM PGCEA
Reflex Zone Therapist, Principal Lecturer in Complementary
Medicine/Midwifery, School of Health, University of Greenwich, London, UK

Forewords by

Denise Rankin-Box BA (Hons) RGN DipTD CertEdMISMA JP
Clinical Specialist in Cardiology; Editor-in-Chief Complementary Therapies in
Nursing and Midwifery

Pat Turton MA MSc RGN FETC
Director of Education, Bristol Cancer Help Centre;
Independent Chair – Reflexology Forum, UK

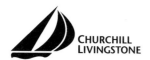
CHURCHILL
LIVINGSTONE

EDINBURGH LONDON NEW YORK OXFORD PHILADELPHIA ST LOUIS SYDNEY TORONTO 2002

CHURCHILL LIVINGSTONE
An imprint of Elsevier Science

First published 2002
  Reprinted 2003

ISBN 0 443 07120 9

British Library Cataloguing in Publication Data
A catalogue record for this book is available from the British Library

Library of Congress Cataloging in Publication Data
A catalog record for this book is available from the Library of Congress

Note
Medical knowledge is constantly changing. As new information
becomes available, changes in treatment, procedures, equipment and
the use of drugs become necessary. The editors, contributors and the
publishers have taken care to ensure that the information given in this
text is accurate and up to date. However, readers are strongly advised
to confirm that the information, especially with regard to drug usage,
complies with the latest legislation and standards of practice.

 your source for books,
journals and multimedia
in the health sciences
www.elsevierhealth.com

The
publisher's
policy is to use
**paper manufactured
from sustainable forests**

Printed in China

Contents

There is a colour plate section at the end of the book

Contributors

M. Denise Tiran MSc RGN RM ADM PGCEA

Denise is Programme Leader for the BSc (Hons) Complementary Therapies and an acknowledged expert on the subject of complementary medicine in maternity care. As a complementary practitioner and practising midwife she runs a busy complementary therapy antenatal clinic at Queen Mary's Hospital, Sidcup, for which she was recently highly commended in the Prince of Wales Awards for Healthcare in London. She has published widely, is a member of the editorial committee of the journal *Complementary Therapies in Nursing and Midwifery* and is a renowned national and international speaker. Denise is Chair of the Complementary Maternity Forum and is currently studying for a PhD. Her chapters on maternity care and on the theories of reflexology draw on her considerable expertise in integrating reflexology and other therapies into clinical practice.

Peter A Mackereth MA RGN CertEd DipNurs DipReflex MCAR AdvReflex (Level3)

Peter has had a varied career in nursing, teaching and research, occupying roles such as Intensive Care Charge Nurse, Nurse Consultant and Research Associate. Peter is currently engaged in a part-time PhD project examining therapeutic outcomes for reflexology. As a practising reflexologist and bodyworker, he works with clients in healthcare settings and private practice. In this book, Peter contributes his experience and understanding of the challenges of integrating this therapy, with particular focus on education, clinical supervision and healing.

Cliff Panton BA CertEd RGN

Cliff has had a varied and rich career in nursing practice and education. As a clinical nurse he has worked mainly in acute settings and as nurse teacher/lecturer has been involved in pre- and post-registration teaching, undergraduate education (mainly complementary therapies and health studies) curriculum design and development and was an Open Learning Project Officer (ENB). In addition to his teaching role, Cliff practises as a clinical reflexologist and therapeutic touch practitioner.

Julie Stone MA LLB

A lecturer in Ethics and Law Applied to Medicine at St Bartholomew's and the London Hospitals, Julie is a lawyer by background and is a recognized expert in the field of ethics, law and regulation of complementary medicine. She was a member of the Regulation Group of the Foundation for Integrated Medicine and advises many complementary and alternative medicine bodies on professional and regulatory issues. She has recently returned from a sabbatical at the University of Hawaii, where she completed her second book (*An Ethical Framework for Complementary and Alternative Therapists*, to be published Routledge, Spring, 2002). She has recently been appointed as a lay member of the GMC. Julie is also training to teach Ashtanga yoga.

Margaret Thorlby RGN Dip(N)Manchester DipReflex AdvReflex (Level3)

Margaret has worked as a nurse for over 10 years, most recently in hospice care. Margaret uses reflexology with patients who have cancer and other life-threatening illnesses. She also contributes regularly to educational programmes on complementary therapies and supervises reflexology students.

Edwina Hodkinson RGN BRCP MAR AdvReflex (Level3) MIFA

Edwina has been a clinical reflexologist for 6 years and has had a busy full-time private practice, which includes work at Bury Hospice, for over 5 years. She has a background in general nursing, working as a sister in general medicine. Edwina is also qualified as a clinical aromatherapist and holds regular courses and workshops on reflexology and cancer care.

Julia M Williams MIGPP MIHAF MAR AOC registered

Julia has been a full-time natural health therapist for the past 10 years. She is a yoga teacher, and holds qualifications in clinical reflexology and aromatherapy, holistic massage, metaphysics, iridology and study of nutrition, together with certificates in counselling skills (health) and teaching in adult education. She was worked with people who have HIV/AIDS, in alcohol rehabilitation, with the elderly (in liaison with Age Concern) and the homeless. For the past 4 years Julia has been a complementary therapist for the haematology directorate at University College London Hospital, working both on the wards and with out-patients.

Clive S O'Hara BRCP MCAR AdvReflex (Level3)

Clive is the Principal Tutor for the Centre for Clinical Reflexology. Clive has been practising reflexology since 1974 and currently teaches reflexology at a number of colleges and higher education institutions. He has contributed to conferences, workshops and television and radio broadcasts on complementary medicine. Clive is a member of the Reflexology Forum and reflexology advisor for the Institute of Complementary Medicine.

to conferences, workshops and television and radio broadcasts on complementary medicine. Clive is a member of the Reflexology Forum and reflexology advisor for the Institute of Complementary Medicine.

Christine Knowles RMN MCAR DipReflex AdvReflex (Level3)

Christine has completed the diploma and advanced reflexology courses with the University of Manchester and Centre for Clinical Reflexology. A registered mental nurse with 13 years' experience in hospitals and the community, Christine has an established private practice and is providing reflexology for a research study at Manchester Royal Infirmary. Christine also provides reflexology, stress management, relaxation and gentle exercise with service users at local drop-in centres for people with mental health needs.

Grace Higgins RMN RGN MCAR DipReflex AdvReflex (Level3)

Grace has completed the diploma and advanced reflexology courses with the University of Manchester and Centre for Clinical Reflexology. Grace has worked in a number of different mental health settings including acute admissions, old age psychiatry and daycare. Currently, Grace is working with people who have multiple sclerosis and chronic fatigue syndrome, and has been part of a community project providing reflexology to people with mental health problems.

Gerry Pyves MA (Oxon) TA(UKCP) DipM (APNT) PGCE

Gerry is an experienced massage therapist with over 20 years in practice. He is one of the UK's most respected teachers on massage, the psychology of touch and the dynamics of the client–practitioner relationship and runs professional development and supervision groups for qualified bodyworkers around the country. He is responsible for the development and dissemination of the 'No Hands' reflexology method.

Helen Poole PhD BSc (Hons)

Helen is a research fellow and part-time lecturer in the School of Health and Human Sciences at Liverpool John Moores University. She has recently completed her doctoral thesis evaluating the use of reflexology for the management of chronic low back pain.

Liz Tipping RM SEN MCAR DipReflex AdvReflex (Level 3)

Liz is an experienced nurse and midwife working on the neonatal intensive care unit at St Mary's Hospital in Manchester. She is qualified in therapeutic touch and reflexology and, in addition to her private practice, is working to incorporate complementary therapies into the care of ill neonates and their parents.

Evelyn Gale PhD MA RCNT RNMH

Evelyn is a Lecturer in Nursing at Keele University, having worked in the field of learning disability for over 20 years. Her experience in complementary therapies is wide and she is qualified in reflexology, massage, aromatherapy and Reiki. The focus for her PhD was an investigation into the use of touch by nurses and its effects on people with a learning disability.

Forewords

It is with pleasure that I write a foreword to *Clinical Reflexology*. This book is a timely and significant resource for anyone who is currently practising or considering using reflexology as a therapeutic tool.

Interest in the practice of reflexology has grown rapidly over the past few years and there is an increasing demand for this therapy in conventional health care settings and in private practice. Alongside this is a need to ensure that practitioners are competent to practice and understand ethicolegal and professional principles as well as issues of safety and efficacy. This book addresses these topics as well as exploring the nature of care through the therapeutic relationship and the application of reflexology in specific fields such as pregnancy and childbirth, palliative care and special needs.

Clinical Reflexology is, perhaps, unique in addressing a broad range of issues associated with this practice. Peter Mackereth and Denise Tiran have drawn upon their own considerable expertise in reflexology and complementary medicine, to create a collaborative venture with contributors also experienced in this field of health care. The result is a text that challenges assumptions underpinning accepted theories and origins of reflexology and offers readers a considered, objective and research based appraisal of this therapy. It also, significantly, introduces innovative clinical techniques.

This book offers an invaluable overview of key issues associated with the practice of reflexology and as such should perhaps be seen as a definitive text on the subject. Indeed, for anyone interested in this therapy, *Clinical Reflexology* is essential reading.

Today, there are many therapies and clinical procedures in complementary and conventional medicine that appear efficacious and yet we do not understand how or why they work. Reflexology is one such practice. This book shows us that when we do not always have the answers we should keep on asking questions, from different perspectives and of different people. In this way we learn and reflect upon our practice.

Much of what we learn in complementary medicine should challenge our world views and perceptions about the nature and effect of the care we give. As we challenge assumptions about the world around us so we too should challenge and explore the rhetoric upon which therapies are based. Simply because a therapy has been practised in a particular way for many years does not necessarily mean it is the most effective way to care for someone. Indeed Gerry Pyves and Peter Mackereth question some of the basic tenets of reflexology by looking at the impact of the therapeutic encounter and draw upon other therapies to consider new techniques in this field such as 'no hands reflexology'. Unless issues such as these are explored, debated and researched, we cannot learn or expand the knowledge base of a therapy. This book then offers us valuable lessons whereby techniques, approaches, theories, reflective practice and of course practitioners themselves, are in a constant state of change. The life experiences a therapist brings to a therapeutic encounter will depend upon what is happening in their own lives and by definition will affect practice. This may not be a bad thing , it is simply something we should be aware of and as this book notes, supervision and support can help us to develop our practice.

I suspect many people practice reflexology and other complementary therapies because what they get out of it is equal to what they put into it. It feels good to help people and the therapeutic encounter is clearly a two way process. If this is not occurring then you have to ask why and try to change practice or attitudes accordingly. Sometimes it is sufficient to not 'do anything' and listen. Improving practice is not always about learning – life remains a struggle whilst one insists it is a struggle – sometimes it is all right to let things unfold. As Margaret Thorlby and Cliff Panton observe, it can be argued that the quality of the therapeutic relationship may be more important than the actual therapy. Thus listening, nurturing and holding touch can be powerful therapeutic tools in themselves.

Peter and Denise have created a text that is indeed more than the sum of its parts. They have developed a tool for working with and developing the practise of reflexology, and they have also produced a text that should cause us to reflect upon the nature of therapeutic care and professional practice. Many issues will also cause you to reflect on other aspects of your life. As Henry Thoreau wrote, 'Many men go fishing all of their lives without knowing that it is not the fish they are after'.

Denise Rankin-Box

We live in a world where an increasing number of people use a range of complementary therapies to help them to manage their illnesses and to promote a sense of wellbeing. People may do this when they feel that orthodox approaches have not yielded sufficiently satisfactory results, sometimes they do it when they have been told that 'nothing further can be done'. We are not necessarily talking here of life-threatening illness, although that may sometimes be the case. More often the problem is the long-standing chronic condition that drains and de-energizes the sufferer, and in the face of which many healthcare professionals feel defeated. Reflexology is one of the most commonly used therapies, which many people find extremely helpful.

Both patients and professionals are frequently surprised by the extent to which people are helped by complementary approaches, and indeed results are sometimes produced which appear to fly in the face of current understanding and accepted medical thinking. Increasingly research begins to unravel complex new theories that emerge from the experiences of patients and the observation of professionals trained in these areas of 'complementary therapies'. The combination of perceived effectiveness, and a growing body of research means that more people are aware of the potential benefits of therapies and wish to access them – either for themselves or, if a healthcare professional, for their patients.

New problems then arise. For the therapists themselves, it is a question of needing a sufficiently high standard of training and education to enable them to meet the expectations and responsibilities that this expanding therapeutic role brings. They also need increased public and professional understanding of their particular therapy, and public and professional confidence in their qualifications and body of knowledge. For patients seeking relief, and for the healthcare professionals who might wish to refer people for appropriate therapies, different issues emerge. What is the nature of the therapy in question? How are they to be sure that the therapists to whom patients may be referred are skilled and trained to an appropriate level?

Currently in the United Kingdom these issues are slowly being addressed. The House of Lords Report of 2000 on Complementary and Alternative Medicine went some way to begin to build a framework for regulation. Bodies such as the Foundation for Integrated Medicine (FIM) are putting a great deal of effort into developing regulatory standards through which the general public and healthcare professionals may be reassured as to whether a particular complementary therapist is appropriately trained and registered. In the case of Reflexology, FIM are promoting this work by supporting the Reflexology Forum. The Forum is a collaborative body of reflexology organizations which work together to promote the professional development of reflexology through the key areas of standards of practice, registration, regulation and education. This is important work, which will serve to safeguard and reassure the public and healthcare professionals. However, although much of the discussion following from the House of Lords report has centred on regulation and registration of complementary and alternative therapies, they are only part of the picture.

At any level where a service is offered to the public, appropriate and adequate training, and an awareness of safe practice are essential.

However, it is one thing to have a complementary therapy as an adjunct to general wellbeing, but it is quite another to provide a service for people who are seeking treatments for the relief of troublesome symptoms, if not indeed actual cure for a range of conditions. Under these circumstances, therapists have a responsibility to undertake a higher level of training and education, to display a greater understanding of the legal and ethical implications and to demonstrate a deeper professional understanding of the application of their therapy in whatever clinical areas they may come to work. They will need to be sure that the knowledge base of their chosen therapy stems from an agreed understanding of the nature of the therapy. They will require an awareness of the research base and associated relevant literature. They should have a clear understanding of the nature of the therapeutic relationship and the implication of this for both patient and therapist.

Education plays a crucial role in the development of the self-aware and skilled professional, whether orthodox of complementary. Both orthodox and complementary practitioners must respect and value the tradition of the other. They must develop a 'shared language' of communication about the issues that concern both. To do this, they need access to appropriate literature provided by experienced practitioners who are themselves educated to a high level. In this way, the knowledge base can be spread, and expanded, and shared with those in other disciplines. The literature can be also be used to provide a sound base for curriculum development at a range of levels.

In many therapies this literature, so essential both to educate and reassure, has been lacking. It is a pleasure therefore, to welcome this new book in the area of clinical reflexology, which provides just such a text as is necessary for the professional development of the advanced practitioner of reflexology. It provides an excellent resource, not only in the material it contains, but also in the clear style and presentation which encourages the reader to reflect on individual cases as well as consider the experimental research base for reflexology, through vignettes, case-studies and extensive and up-to-date references. An additional valuable feature of the book is that the chapters are provided by a range of contributors each of whom are skilled in their particular area. Hence it is not the product of one single reflexology organization, and this promotes the development of a knowledge base that can be said to underpin the profession as a whole.

I am privileged to have been appointed Independent Chair of the Reflexology Forum, and in that capacity I am aware of the need for texts such as this to support the education programmes of clinical reflexology. In my work as Director of Education and Development at the Bristol Cancer Help Centre, I work not only with service providers, but also with a range of educational institutions. In this work I frequently encounter barriers to integration that good and clear text books can help to break down. In addition, I look to complementary therapists to provide appropriate texts that can be used for the education of their fellow therapists in more specialist clinical areas. I particularly welcome, therefore, this helpful contribution to the literature supporting and developing the practice of clinical reflexology.

Pat Turton

Preface

As practitioners of reflexology, members of the conventional healthcare professions and university lecturers in complementary medicine, we perceived a need for a text on reflexology that would enable others to explore the nature, status and potential of this fascinating therapy. Numerous reflexology texts are available, written by experienced and enthusiastic practitioners who have seen the benefits of treating clients in private practice. In contrast, many of the ideas in this new book have evolved from the process and challenges of integrating theory and practice, as well as using reflexology in the National Health Service.

Students on university degree programmes are also driving the demand for high quality, research-based and accessible texts to supplement their classroom and clinical learning. Equally, clients require their therapists to utilize contemporary information to support their practice, so that they can be reassured of an individualized, effective yet safe service.

It is inevitable, in the pursuit of greater integration of complementary therapies into conventional healthcare, that reflexology (and other therapies) will evolve and will need to be adapted to meet the needs of the system in which it finds itself. However, there is also a need to identify and retain the valuable core principles of the original therapy and ensure that these are not lost in the process. Similarly, it is essential to acquire a deeper understanding of the theory of the therapy to explore further its place and increasing credibility in modern health care. It behoves the profession of reflexology to produce critical and reflective practitioners, and to acknowledge the value of research and enquiry in this process.

In preparing this text we were concerned to communicate and disseminate our understanding and appraisal of the therapy at this time, in order to encourage others to debate objectively so as to enhance the development of the profession. This book, therefore, has a strong focus on key professional issues such as accountability, legal and ethical concerns and health and safety issues. These aspects are developed further in Section 2, in which the chapters are dedicated to specialist areas of clinical practice and are illustrated with case scenarios drawn from the experience of the contributors.

The contributors are involved in a variety of professional activities related to complementary medicine, including practice, research, teaching and publication. They are respected colleagues and fellow learners in the art and science of reflexology and, as editors, we would like to extend our thanks to them all for their motivation and enthusiasm during the preparation of the book.

In selecting this book for your studies we feel that you are entering into a journey of exploration and discovery. We hope it will go some way towards inspiring you to continue your learning so that you attain your personal potential as a creative reflexologist and are motivated to engage in the challenge of acquiring the necessary evidence for increased integration and to act as a role model for others within the profession.

Denise Tiran

2002 Peter Mackereth

Acknowledgements

The Editors would like to thank all the contributors who have worked tirelessly to bring this work to fruition, especially in the light of all the other personal and professional issues in their lives. Special thanks to all the clients and patients whose (anonymous) case scenarios have served to illuminate elements of the text.

Denise would like to give a big hug to her 12-year-old son, Adam, for all the evenings and weekends she was unable to spend with him, as well as colleagues at the University of Greenwich and Queen Mary's Hospital, Sidcup, who have, as ever, been immensely supportive.

Peter would like to thank Stephen McGinn for his unstinting technological support and cups of Earl Grey tea, and patients and colleagues at Manchester Royal Infirmary and Christie Hospital.

Key themes in Clinical Reflexology: A Guide for Health Professionals

---

SECTION CONTENTS

Introduction

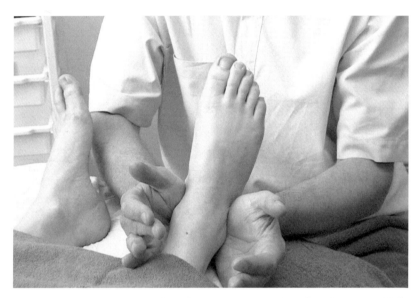

Photo courtesy of Katie Spruce BA (Hons), medical photographer, Christie Hospital NHS Trust, with permission.

This book on clinical reflexology has been divided into two sections. The first section consists of eight chapters, each a critical review of a contemporary theme related to clinical reflexology by authors with specific expertise on the topics. Deciding which areas to focus on emerged from the editors' experience of providing reflexology in healthcare settings, teaching and supervising students of reflexology, and participating in research work. It is important for the reader to be aware that the contents of the book unfold progressively, with the themes in Section 1 providing a foundation for the examination of clinical reflexology practice that is the focus of Section 2.

All chapters begin with a short abstract and key words. The authors have included useful supportive references, integration of case studies and a list of further resources and reading.

Chapter 1. Reviewing the theories and origins by Denise Tiran. This chapter provides a critical review of the theories and origins of reflexology.

Its purpose is to present the reader with an appraisal of these rather than to propound one stance.

Chapter 2. Appreciating preparatory and continuing education by Peter Mackereth and Clive O'Hara. The authors of this chapter are teachers, supervisors and practitioners of clinical reflexology. They have written a critical review of the education and regulation issues related to pre-registration programmes, continuing education and practice development.

Chapter 3. Challenging the 'rules' of reflexology by Clive O'Hara. After debating and challenging the 'rules' for practice, Clive O'Hara considers how a more flexible approach might be beneficial for healthcare in general and could facilitate the incorporation of reflexology as a viable therapeutic intervention within conventional healthcare.

Chapter 4. Identifying ethicolegal and professional principles by Julie Stone. Ethical and legal responsibilities are integral to safe and effective practice. Written by a lawyer and lecturer in ethics and law, this chapter outlines the major ethical and legal responsibilities owed by reflexologists to their patients.

Chapter 5. Researching reflexology by Helen Poole. The author of this chapter is a researcher who has conducted a doctoral study of reflexology. Here, she explores the issue of research within the reflexology profession, suggests what questions should be asked and makes some suggestions for the direction of future research. A review of some of the published reflexology research is also included.

Chapter 6. Clarifying healing and holism by Peter Mackereth. This chapter explores definitions of healing and holism and how these terms relate to the clinical practice of reflexology. The concepts of spirituality and the phenomena of the 'healing crisis', referred to in many reflexology texts, are examined. Important issues related to the role of practitioner, the therapeutic relationship and the space in which the interaction takes place are also explored.

Chapter 7. Exploring the therapeutic relationship by Cliff Panton and Margaret Thorlby. The therapeutic relationship as an essential part of reflexology treatment is explored in this chapter. The authors also consider the quality of the relationship within the therapeutic milieu and the concepts of partnership and empowerment as essential components of a proposed model for clinical reflexology.

Chapter 8. Practising safely and effectively by Gerry Pyves and Peter Mackereth. Using an approach developed by Gerry Pyves, called 'No Hands' reflexology, the authors explore the concept of performing reflexology to avoid injury to the therapist and to re-evaluate conventional reflexology techniques. The chapter includes postural recommendations and adaptation techniques. The authors also briefly identify and discuss other key issues related to the practice of clinical reflexology (some of which are explored more fully in other chapters).

1

Reviewing theories and origins

Denise Tiran

Abstract

There are many theories about how and why reflexology is thought to work, some more recent than others. This chapter reviews some of the current literature regarding the processes of reflexology, but does not attempt to come to a definitive conclusion.

Key words: historical perspectives, theories and charts

Reflexology is the use of a sophisticated system of touch, usually on the feet, but sometimes on the hands, ears, face, tongue or back, in which the area being massaged is thought to correspond to a map of the whole body. In this way, working on specific areas of the feet can influence other areas of the body, while a full treatment is, in effect, a full body massage. Reflexology is, however, not simply a massage but is also a powerful system of health care, useful for achieving and maintaining health and enhancing wellbeing, as well as for relieving symptoms or causes of illness and disease. It is expounded as a means of maintaining homeostasis, aiding relaxation and triggering the body's own innate self-healing capacity (Lett 2000).

Experienced reflexologists are also able to identify from the feet areas of the body that are affected by changing physiology or current, previous or impending pathology, although the therapy should not truly be considered as a diagnostic technique; this will be discussed further later in this chapter and by Clive O'Hara in Chapter 3. By inference, it should be possible to prevent impending illness from occurring, or at least to reduce its severity.

ORIGINS OF REFLEXOLOGY

It is thought that reflexology has been used in some form or other since ancient times, for there is evidence in various cultures of different types of foot treatment being carried out. These have been found in India, from over 5000 years BC, in Assyria and in Egypt, from paintings in a physician's tomb of 2500 BC (although modern-day Egyptologists debate whether the pictographs show a foot massage, a pedicure or a surgical procedure). The Chinese may have used it as long ago as 4000 BC and foot treatment is documented by the Yellow Emperor who died in 2598 BC (Issel 1993, cited by Enzer 2000). Traditional Chinese medicine has long recognized a link between one part of the body and another in order to appreciate the whole being, and works on the theory that disorder or disease in one area will disrupt the whole person. Indeed, Turgeon (1994) suggests that auriculotherapy is a form of ear reflexology, although it is more commonly considered to be ear acupuncture. Similarly, Crane (1997), who has been instrumental in returning the practice of reflexology to the Chinese in recent years, acknowledges ear reflexology and categorically links the origins of the therapy to Chinese meridians (see below).

More recently, at the beginning of the twentieth century, the American ear, nose and throat specialist, William Fitzgerald, discovered that Native American Indians used foot treatment, passing information down through generations by word of mouth. As a result of his investigations he began to advocate a compression technique of the fingers for pain relief in patients undergoing minor maxillofacial surgery. He identified ten longitudinal zones in the body, five on each side of the midline, running from the toes and fingers to the head, which appeared to correspond to other areas of the body. Fitzgerald is acknowledged to be the founder of modern zone therapy and worked in collaboration with colleagues in medicine, dentistry and osteopathy.

In the 1930s, an American masseuse, Eunice Ingham, started to use Fitzgerald's work as a basis for further refinement of the therapy and finished the process of mapping the feet to reflect the zones of the whole body. She developed a special system of compression massage of the feet, sometimes called 'thumb walking' (Enzer 2000) or the particularly descriptive 'caterpillar crawling' (Wagner 1987).

One of Ingham's students, Doreen Bayly, brought the treatment to Europe and established the first school of reflexology in the UK. In Germany a nurse, Hanne Marquardt, exploring Fitzgerald's longitudinal zones further, imposed three transverse zones on the feet. She created a more sophisticated zone chart with additional reflex zones on the dorsum of the foot and the sole, and the therapy became known as reflex zone therapy. Numerous schools of reflex zone therapy were established throughout Europe. Additional work by Froneberg led to the recognition of reflex zones to the nervous system and musculature, leading to an adapted form of treatment called manual neurotherapy for use on people with impaired neural pathways (cited by Lett 2000).

Reflexology, reflex zone therapy or reflexotherapy are all terms that refer to the current use of the treatment, distinctions apparently being due to scientific, philosophical, political or commercial differences of opinion between authorities.

Adapted forms of the therapy include the Morrell method, developed by Pat Morrell in Wales, and the similar holistic multidimensional system, both of which involve extremely gentle pressure and result in therapeutic benefit with a minimal healing crisis (Griffiths 2000). The Metamorphic technique focuses specifically on the foot zones for the spine, which are thought to correspond to the 9 months of intrauterine life; early treatment on these zones can prevent any exacerbation of problems that could have been triggered in gestational life. Two more recent forms of reflexology are the commercially viable 'vacuflex' system, which combines reflexology, acupressure and the cupping technique of traditional Chinese medicine, and upright reflexology, in which the dorsum of each foot is treated with the client standing upright.

REFLEXOLOGY CHARTS

Reflexologists learn about the therapy and the areas of the feet that correspond to other parts of the body from 'maps', or charts, most of which are based on a reiteration or mirror image of the body. Reflex zone therapy additionally uses longitudinal and horizontal zones within the body. There are, however, several types of charts, each one slightly different from the others.

REITERATIVE CHARTS

These use zones and the maps reflect the whole body in miniature superimposed on a diagram of a foot, so that the therapist can identify which part of the foot refers to which specific area of the body. These are the most commonly used charts, particularly in Western reflexology, although there may be minor variations between those of different authorities.

EMPIRICAL CHARTS

These are more individual and are devised from an accumulation of personal experience by one or more practitioners, but these can vary widely from the more standard charts. From a slightly cynical commercial viewpoint, many of these charts are covered by copyright regulations and are often included in textbooks written by the different authorities wishing to make or maintain a reputation.

CHINESE TRADITIONAL CHARTS

These use the theory of a link with acupuncture meridians but do not necessarily correspond to the reiterative charts, although, as mentioned previously, many reflexology points correspond to *tsubos* used in acupuncture.

ARTISTIC CHARTS

These are produced to be visually appealing and often contain inaccuracies; they should not be relied upon for practitioner use. Unfortunately, current interest in all aspects of complementary and alternative medicine has resulted in the production of numerous colourful charts, as wall posters: one of the most inaccurate seen by this author was actually included as an insert in a popular weekly nursing magazine.

ANCIENT CHARTS

These can be found in Asia, although Kunz & Kunz (1998) question whether the ancient pictographs are indeed old charts. In any case, much of the original meaning has been lost or misinterpreted over the ages.

THEORIES TO EXPLAIN HOW REFLEXOLOGY WORKS

There would be no valid reason for considering *how* reflexology works if we did not know (or have some supposition) *whether* it works. *If* the therapy has some effect, whether it is physiological, psychological or spiritual, then we need to ask first, *what* does it do? and only second, *how* does it work?

That reflexology actually does *something* is undoubted, although the effects may not necessarily be immediately perceived by the client or therapist. On some occasions it may be the client's relatives who recognize that they are more relaxed. Even the family dog may react differently to the client post-treatment! However, frequently during and immediately following treatment clients have variously reported experiencing reactions such as localized or distal pain, perspiration or shivering, changes in heart rate, respiration or temperature, nausea or emotional upheavals (Marquardt 2000). Every practitioner will have witnessed some or all of these responses in their clients, but although textbooks include accounts of expected reactions to treatment, there is little evidence recorded in the research literature.

Small-scale research trials on healthy volunteers have examined physiological effects, demonstrated via ultrasonography, such as changes in the renal blood flow. A study by Sudmeier et al (1999) has been acknowledged as providing 'good supportive evidence' for reflexology (White 1999). However, other trials, for example, Frankel's (1997) investigation of the effect on baroreceptors, blood pressure and sinus arrhythmia, Shirley et al's exploration of neurophysiological effects (undated) and Zhigin's (undated) report on gall bladder constriction, do not stand up to such rigorous scrutiny.

A range of theories as to how reflexology works has been put forward by various authorities. However, the somewhat incestuous nature of contemporary reflexology, in Europe in particular, means that much of the earlier information has been passed down as accepted fact and collated by a few specialists, who then place their own interpretation and bias on the detail, with little prior evidence of its accuracy.

Vast numbers of relatively recent reflexology research reports originate from China, but they generally use small cohorts of subjects, are rarely randomized, double-blinded or controlled, often contain multiple confounding variables and may also lose some of their meaning in the translation to English. Many of the authors of these reports also seem to make sweeping assumptions about their findings. This is not to say that the Chinese research should be dismissed, but in order for it to gain acceptance in conventional medical circles it needs to be published in recognized journals rather than in the non-peer-reviewed newsletters and websites of individual schools and organizations of reflexology. On the other hand we should not assume that the 'gold standard' randomized controlled trial (RCT) is the only way to demonstrate effectively the value of any complementary therapy, however, its use does eliminate some of the potential monopoly on ownership of knowledge and helps to add credibility in the eyes of the medical professions.

There are, however, a few theories that can be substantiated and understood via conventional principles. Fitzgerald attempted to explain to his medical colleagues the actions of reflex zone therapy by its analgesic, relaxation and nerve blocking effects, as well as by the induction of relative venous stasis in the zone corresponding to the affected area (Crane 1997, Marquardt 2000).

Indeed, one of the actions of reflexology may be attributed to the *gate control theory*, an accepted mechanism to explain pain control, first recognized by Melzack & Wall (1965) and on which analgesia such as transcutaneous electrical nerve stimulation (TENS) is thought to work. Reflexology may work similarly to a TENS machine, relieving or suppressing pain impulses. This may be similar to the impact of any touch therapy, for it is known that touch impulses reach the brain before pain impulses, thereby effectively 'shutting the gate' to the perception of pain.

Alternatively, reflexology may work by *stimulating the release of endorphins and encephalins*, the body's natural pain relievers and mood enhancers. Generalized massage and touch therapies have frequently been found to reduce the perception of pain through this mechanism (Day et al 1987, Ferrell-Torry & Glick 1993, Ginsberg & Famey 1987, Kaada & Torsteinbo 1989).

These two theories may be more in keeping with a 'Western' approach to health care than some of those that follow, as they are demonstrable and conceivable. Similarly, the placebo effect and the client–therapist relationship (see Chapter 7) may be more significant in affecting health outcomes than the actual type of treatment. It is well known that interactions between clients and their healthcare practitioners, both complementary and conventional, can influence health outcomes positively or negatively, irrespective of the impact of treatment on the specific disease or condition. The effect on clients/patients of being listened to and receiving continuity of care from an individual practitioner goes a long way towards making them feel valued, which in turn helps them to feel 'better'. Crane (1997) disagrees that 'positive results' are solely due to client expectation but offers no evidence to support her view or any suggestions for an alternative hypothesis.

The *relaxation effect* of the treatment may also help to reduce or relieve stress, thus preventing or alleviating illnesses triggered by stress, for example, hypertension. This could, however, be due simply to the effect of touch, rather than anything specific to reflexology, for massage has been shown to increase wellbeing and relaxation (Farrow 1990, Field et al 1993, Fraser & Kerr 1993, McKechnie et al 1983, Sims 1986). Treatment is known to induce in some clients a deep fatigue and a desire to rest and sleep, which in itself may be an opportunity for the body to recoup its energy.

More controversial ideas have come to the fore recently. For example, *electromagnetic theories* about how reflexology works are based on the belief that the human brain, in common with other organic matter, vibrates and emits alpha waves, measurable on an electroencephalogram. Similarly, the earth vibrates at a rate comparable with alpha brain waves; this is called Schuman resonance. The brain is considered to be the link between the vibrations of the earth and our bodies; if the brain vibrates at an alpha rhythm a person should be in equilibrium with his or her surroundings and thus in good health. Bliss & Bliss (1999) liken the brain to a radio transmitter sending and receiving electromagnetic messages to regulate the frequency of the vibrations. However, at times of physical or emotional stress these messages can become distorted or blocked, or the vibrational rate may be reduced. Healing with reflexology may occur as a result of 'sympathetic resonance', whereby the alpha waves of the healer are transmitted to the client, assisting in the process of restoring homeostasis. It is postulated that the 'grounding' that many therapists undertake prior to treatment increases the link between the earth's vibrational energy and that of the practitioner.

Bliss & Bliss (1999) state that fluctuations in electromagnetic energy of healers have been demonstrated, with a substantial difference in measured biomagnetic energy in the hands during treatment, compared to other areas of the body, notably the brain and heart. They suggest that around

7 Hz of energy may be transmitted from the hands of the therapist, possibly facilitating healing of different types of tissue within the body. However, no references are given to support this information. On a simple level, many practitioners report feeling a sense of relaxation when undertaking treatments, possibly indicating a two-way transmission of energy between client and therapist.

Lett (2000) reminds us of the discovery of the reflex signs of disease and the impact of illness in one part of the body on another distal area, for example, the shoulder pain experienced with problems of the gall bladder. The *nerve impulse theory* (Bliss & Bliss 2000) is based on the principle that pressure to the foot (or other areas) triggers afferent neurons to convey messages to the brain via the ganglia and spinal cord. The fingers and toes are particularly sensitive to touch and pressure because of their large number of Meissner's receptors, which carry touch impulses to the brain, and of Pacinian corpuscles, which convey pressure impulses. Messages are returned via the motor neurons, spinal cord and ganglia to the relevant muscle groups. Reflexology is thought to work directly on the muscles as a result of a combining of the messages coming from the feet with those going to the muscles. Kunz & Kunz (1998) refer to this as the *autonomic–somatic integration theory*, in which reflexology assists with the stress mechanism, the autonomic, somatic and motor nervous systems. Lett (2000) also subscribes to the neural pathway approach and cites research by Baldry (1998) in which it has been suggested that stimulation of dermal and muscular nociceptors triggers messages of pain and that this can be suppressed by needle stimulation of mechanothermal receptors, thus activating encephalinergic inhibitory interneurons in the dorsal horn. This may also give support to the meridian theory (see below).

The *energy flow theory* suggests that positive and negative energy receptors in the feet connect with those in the ground. Congestion within the feet affects their ability to pick up energy from the earth so that the flow of energy is impeded; reflexology enables an unblocking of impeded energy and allows the feet to regain their links with the ground energy. This theory does not, however, explain adequately why hand, ear or face reflexology should be effective. The *proprioceptive theory* is similar in that it supports the spatial relationship of the feet with the ground.

The *meridian theory* is one of the most popular and appears to have been gaining more ground in recent years. It is based on the ancient Chinese system of meridians, channels of subtle energy, called *Qi*, which flow through the body from top to toe, often following the line of a neural pathway. When the body, mind and spirit are in equilibrium the energy flows unimpeded along the meridians, but disease or disorder, stress or pain can result in energy changes, including excessive or inadequate *Qi*, or stagnation. Reflexology is one means of rebalancing the *Qi* by unblocking, stimulating or sedating the energy flow. Crane (1997) explores the relationship between reflexology and acupuncture points in detail and suggests that it is often the distal points on a meridian that are most therapeutically effective, namely those situated in the hands and feet, which correspond to reflexology points. Many of the known reflexology points on the feet and hands correlate to *tsubos*, the acupuncture points used in traditional Chinese medicine, for example, the solar plexus zone corresponds to kidney 1, a point in the middle of the plantar surface of the foot, used to achieve relaxation. Lett (2000) refers to the extracellular matrix of the body's connective tissues and the ground-regulating system, to which she attributes the analgesic actions of both reflexology and acupuncture.

However, it is inaccurate and misleading to describe reflexology as acupressure because much of the pressure used during reflexology or reflex zone therapy is not applied to the *tsubos* used in acupressure/acupuncture. Although clinical combination of different therapies may work synergistically, the theories of each therapy should remain separate unless and until there is sufficient research evidence to support their combination. In the words of Ursula James (2001), Director of the London College of Clinical Hypnotherapy: 'fusion is applaudable, but confusion is deplorable'(personal communication).

Kunz & Kunz (1998) cite research by a Chinese physicist and his colleagues, Cho (undated), working in the US, who discovered an MRI image correlation between needling of eye-related acupuncture points on the feet and shining a light in the eyes. In addition, there were other differences in the MRI-measured brain activity of the twelve volunteers in the study, which the acupuncturists attributed to yin and yang energies. It was thought that, as nerves in the feet connect to the central nervous system and the section of the brain that includes the visual cortex, acupuncture signals may stimulate the hypothalamus, thereby releasing neurochemicals, which, together with the autonomic nervous system, may benefit disorders of the vision.

Bliss & Bliss (1999) also refer to a '*feet as the U bend theory*', in which, because the feet are the furthest point away from the heart, and the point at which gravitational effects are most significant, they act in principle like the U bend in a plumbing system. Serum deposits of calcium and uric acid are thought to build up in the feet, often felt as gravel-like deposits under the skin in the zone of the foot corresponding to the affected area of the body. This has also been termed the *lactic acid theory*, which has now been largely rejected in favour of others. Reflexology is thought to break down and disperse these deposits, allowing the body's energy to recirculate, thus improving blood and lymph flow and returning the body to homeostasis. Marquardt (2000), however, makes no mention of this in relation to reflex zone therapy/reflexotherapy.

Frandsen (1998) favours the *embryo containing information of the whole organism (ECIWO) theory*, in which the human body has, in evolutionary terms, lost the ability to generate a whole new person from one detached part, unlike some lower organisms, yet we have retained the capacity to self-heal since embryonic times. Thus each part holds information of the whole and the human body consists of ECIWOs at different levels, the feet being at a relatively high level, with the left and right foot each representing half of the body. In this way, a map or chart can be drawn which outlines the whole body in miniature across both feet. This theory does lend weight to the use of other areas of the body for reflexology, such as the hand, ear, face or back, as well as auricular acupuncture, iridology and Chinese tongue and facial diagnosis, based on the principle of ECIWOs in each separate body part. Frandsen (1998), a Danish practitioner, confirms that reflexology is generally concerned primarily with the feet and is now more commonly termed reflex therapy of the feet. However, he proposes a new definition for reflexology, which identifies it as: 'the therapeutic application of the fact that delimited parts of an organism correspond to the whole organism' (Frandsen 1998).

REFLEXOLOGY AS A DIAGNOSTIC TOOL

It is generally held that there is a two-way relationship between the feet and the rest of the body. In this way, disorders in the body are reflected in the feet and disorders of the feet reflect the condition of the body. It is not intended that reflexology should be used, in the conventional sense, as a discrete tool for making a diagnosis. Indeed, although there is no legal restriction in the UK on complementary practitioners diagnosing, Napoleonic law in Europe prohibits anyone other than a medically qualified doctor from making a diagnosis.

However, it is possible to elicit signs from the feet from which a skilled practitioner can deduce possible or actual physiopathology in a specific area of the body. These signs might be changes in the tone, colour or shape of a particular area of one or both feet so that an educated guess can be made about the client's condition. Experience will assist the practitioner in defining whether the problem is current, acute, chronic, an old resolved condition or one that is just developing. The experienced therapist will also be able to differentiate between changing physiology or actual pathology, for example, the difference between normal gastrointestinal activity or a possible problem of the digestive tract.

Deciding on a 'diagnosis' may be influenced by a piecing together of the history of the client with intuition and experience of the therapist. A comprehensive examination of the feet at the start of a series of treatments can be very revealing and clients are frequently amazed at what the therapist is able to deduce about their state of health. Stormer (1995) and Enzer (2000) suggest that, in addition to the identification of previous, current or impending disease, examination of the feet can elicit the psychological wellbeing of the person as well as specific personality traits. Each foot reflects different qualities of the whole person, such as internal and external energy, practical and creative aspects, feminine and masculine components and these can be used to identify those people more at risk of certain conditions as a result of their personality. Crane (1997) also utilizes astrological signs as a predictor of health, mapping the signs on diagrams of the feet over the zones corresponding to those areas of the body in which they are more at risk of disorders or disease.

However, reflexology is a holistic therapy that aims to treat the whole person. As a result of this philosophy many practitioners hold the view that they do not need to make a diagnosis, as a whole treatment will treat the whole person, irrespective of the causes or effects of the illness. This is an irresponsible attitude in an age when complementary medicine is attempting to become better integrated alongside conventional health care. Diagnosis, in its broadest sense, involves identification of what reflexologists can treat and what is outside the scope of their practice. It is not appropriate to treat every client/patient the same so it is necessary to confirm what is different about each client in order to perform the most therapeutic techniques and give the most appropriate advice.

Conversely, reflex zone therapy can be extremely effective when used in a more reductionist manner, along the lines of conventional treatments, by working on foot or hand zones corresponding only to the affected part of the body. Purists will dispute this as it takes no account of the causative links within the body, simply relieving symptoms or easing pain and discomfort. Similarly, they will disagree with the controversial concept of combining therapies, for example, using aromatherapy essential oils to complete a treatment, although experience of this author suggests that they work synergistically for the overall benefit of the client.

CONCLUSION

This chapter has considered some of the traditional and more contemporary (and at times controversial) theories regarding the mode of action and the effects of reflexology. The debate is by no means exhausted; indeed it may only just be beginning. It is vital that, in order to develop further as a discrete profession, reflexology practitioners continue to explore these theories, and to challenge long-held 'facts' that have been passed down from one person to the next. It is hoped that this chapter has set the scene for some of the issues discussed in the following chapters and that it will motivate and stimulate readers to pursue the debate further.

REFERENCES

Baldry PE. Trigger point acupuncture. In: Filshie J, White A, eds. Medical acupuncture: a Western scientific approach. New York: Churchill Livingstone; 1998.

Bliss J, Bliss G. How does reflexology work? Theories on why it does work. Reflexology Association of California. On-line. Available: http://www.reflexcal.org/article4.html 15 February 2000.

Cho Z-H. Cited by Kunz K, Kunz B. Groundbreaking research in acupuncture to impact reflexology. On-line. Available: http://www.reflexology-research.com/mri.htm 15 February 2000.

Crane B. Reflexology: the definitive practitioner's manual. Shaftesbury, Dorset: Element; 1997.

Day JA, Mason RR, Chesrow SE. Effect of massage on serum level beta-endorphins and beta-lipotropin in healthy adults. Physical Therapy 1987; 67(6):926–930.

Enzer S. Reflexology: a tool for midwives. Australia: self-published; 2000.

Farrow J. Massage therapy and nursing care. Nursing Standard 1990; 4(17):26–28.

Ferrell-Torry AT, Glick OJ. The use of therapeutic massage as a nursing intervention to modify anxiety and the perception of cancer pain. Cancer Nursing 1993; 16(2):93–101.

Field T, Morrow C, Vaideon C, et al. Massage reduces anxiety in child and adolescent psychiatric patients. International Journal of Alternative and Complementary Medicine 1993; 11(7):22–27.

Frandsen PL. Why does reflexology work? – Is the explanation found in the embryo? Denmark: FDZ; 1998.

Frankel BSM. The effect of reflexology on baroreceptor reflex sensitivity, blood pressure and sinus arrhythmia. Complementary Therapies in Medicine 1997; 5:80–84.

Fraser J, Kerr JR. Psychophysiogical effects of back massage on elderly institutionalised patients. Journal of Advanced Nursing 1993; 18:238–245.

Ginsberg F, Famey JP. A double-blind study of topical massage with Rado-salil ointment in mechanical low back pain. Journal of International Medical Research 1987; 15:148–153.

Griffiths P. Reflexology. In Rankin-Box D, ed. The Nurses' Handbook of Complementary Therapies. 2nd edn. 241–248. London: Harcourt Publishers Ltd; 2001.

Kaada B, Torsteinbo O. Increase of plasma beta-endorphins in connective tissue massage. General Pharmacology 1989; 20(4):487–489.

Kunz K, Kunz B. Ground breaking research in acupuncture to impact reflexology. On-line. Available: http://www.reflexology-research.com/howto.html 9 January 1998.

Lett A. Reflex zone therapy for health professionals. London: Churchill Livingstone; 2000.

McKechnie AA, Wilson F, Watson N, Scott D. Anxiety states: a preliminary report on the value of connective tissue massage. Journal of Psychosomatic Research 1983; 27(2):125–129.

Marquardt H. Reflexotherapy of the feet. Stuttgart: Thieme; 2000.

Melzack R, Wall PD. Pain mechanisms: a new theory. Science 1965; 150:971–979.

Shirley C, Young M, Ackland T, Thompson PM. Effects of reflexology on neurophysiological functioning. In: White A, ed. Reflexology research record 1999; Exeter: University of Exeter.

Sims S. Slow stroke back massage for cancer patients. Nursing Times 1986; 82(13):47–50.

Stormer C. The language of the feet. London: Heinemann; 1995.

Sudmeier I, Bodner G, Egger I et al. Changes of the renal blood flow during organ-associated foot reflexology measured by colour Doppler sonography. Forschende Komplementarmedizin 1999; 6(3):129–134.

Turgeon M. Right brain, left brain reflexology. (Translated by Guoin MA from the original Turgeon M La reflexologie du cerveau pour auditifs et vissels. Quebec: Editions de Montagne; 1988.) Vermont: Healing Arts Press; 1994.

Wagner F. Reflex zone massage. London: Thorsons; 1987.

White A. Reflexology research record (prepared for the Reflexology Research Trust). Exeter: Department of Complementary Medicine, University of Exeter; 1999.

Zhigin D (undated) Observation of constriction effect on normal human gallbladder induced by foot reflex zone massage. In: Reflexology Research Reports. London: Association of Reflexologists; undated. London.

2

Appreciating preparatory and continuing education

Peter A Mackereth and Clive S O'Hara

Abstract

The increasing interest in reflexology by healthcare professionals clearly demonstrates an awakening to its healing potential and is signalled by the demand for texts such as this. There is also interest in pursuing and providing educational programmes within universities and other Higher Education (HE) institutions (Faltermeyer 1995, Nicholl 1995). The majority of reflexologists have completed vocational training, provided largely by the private sector and local further education colleges and commonly approved by reflexology regulation bodies with established assessment policies and procedures. This chapter was prompted by the experience of teaching students studying reflexology at academic level 2 (diploma) and 3 (undergraduate). These students are expected to utilize the literature and, although reflexology-specific articles and textbooks are increasing in number and improving in quality, they often lack the level of critical analysis required by students and teachers. There is a need to recognize that reflexology is making strides to produce 'fit-for-purpose' practitioners able to offer their skills in an ever-widening practice arena. An important measure of professionalism is an assurance that practitioners maintain and improve their work for the benefit of their clients. The aim of this chapter, then, is to review the education and regulation issues related to pre-registration programmes and to look at the approaches to continuing education and practice development.

Key words: professionalism, competence, self-regulation, continuing education, supervision

The last few decades have seen a phenomenal growth in the interest in complementary therapies from both the general public and healthcare professions. For example, in nursing this has led to the emergence of a specialist interest group within the Royal College of Nursing and midwives have established the Complementary Maternity Forum. Healthcare journals are increasingly including papers on complementary and alternative medicine

(CAM) topics and, more recently, CAM journals and textbooks have been published aimed at healthcare professionals. Reflexology has become one of the most common therapies practised by nurses and midwives in the UK (Rankin-Box 1997). This movement has produced leaders in promoting the integration, teaching and research of reflexology in clinical practice. Partnerships that have evolved between practitioners working in the private and public healthcare sectors have provided opportunities to exchange ideas and broaden the use of reflexology in such areas as mental health and palliative care (see Section 2 and specialist practice areas). Patients are asking for their reflexologists to provide treatments while they are in hospital, and at the same time nurses and midwives are clearly learning the skills to provide treatments themselves (Dryden et al 1998, Tiran 1996). It is important to examine how practitioners currently develop skills in reflexology and to identify the key issues in developing the profession for work in conventional healthcare settings.

Education and training in reflexology has improved over the past few years from what has been described as a 'cottage industry' (Cant & Sharma 1996) led by energetic and committed practitioners. There are currently in excess of 13 reflexology groups and associations in the UK, and hundreds worldwide, some representing graduates from only one school. This situation can be a 'minefield' for members of the public looking for independent information about practitioners or courses. As there is no legislation formally regulating reflexology practice in the UK, anyone can refer to himself or herself as a reflexologist, and establish and advertise their business (see Chapter 4). The only safeguard to the public is that in order to obtain professional indemnity insurance practitioners have to produce proof of qualification, known to be of a standard that is of satisfaction to the insurer. However, there will always be people who are willing to risk practising without insurance or may not appreciate the importance of protecting their clients and their practice. There are also self-taught individuals who are offering reflexology for monetary gain without any external assessment or monitoring of their skills. Others have completed an adult education course intended as a 'taster' or for non-commercial use with family and friends. Before examining the current and future developments in the preparation and supervision of practitioners it is important to examine the recent past.

LEARNING FROM THE PAST

Most textbooks are informative about the Egyptian, Chinese, Oriental and American Indian and, more lately, European evidence that reflexology is rooted in history. Literature adequately explaining the relationship between zone theory and the meridians of acupuncture and the influence of Fitzgerald, Bowers and Riley abounds. Eunice Ingham is considered by the majority to be the 'true matriarch' of Western reflexology (Adamson et al 1995). The training organization established by Ingham and her nephew, Dwight C Byers, was the route by which most British reflexology pioneers came into practice and it would therefore seem appropriate to start with her. Eunice Ingham has been referred to as a physiotherapist, a massage therapist and an assistant to, or pupil of, Joseph Riley (Adamson et al 1995, Dougans 1996, Gore 1990, Norman 1988), and so could also be referred to as the first reflexologist with a conventional health professional background. Ingham shared her findings and resulting zone maps with other professionals in the orthodox and complementary medical fields (such as chiropodists, naturopaths, masseurs and physiotherapists) and wrote four books. Ingham was most successful in the US with training lay practitioners and instructing the public in self-help and treating family and friends (Adamson et al 1995). Since Eunice Ingham's death in 1974, the International Institute of Reflexology has exclusive rights to teach worldwide her original method of reflexology, which is presided over by Dwight C Byers. As with all groundbreaking ideas, it took individuals with great strength of character and determination to introduce reflexology training into their own country.

Doreen Bayly has been credited as the person who brought reflexology practice and training into the UK. When living in the US Doreen trained with Ingham, and then returned to the UK and established the first British training school in 1968 (Hall 1997). Bayly is not the only one to be instrumental in awakening the interest of the British public in reflexology. Ann Gillanders, who in 1973 trained with Dwight C Byers, along with her brother Anthony Porter were also early pioneers of reflexology in the UK in the 1970s. In 1979 Gillanders took over the directorship of the International Institute of Reflexology, the training organization for the 'Ingham method', and in 1986 established the Holistic Healing Centre, the base of the British School of Reflexology.

Robert Dallamore, a Londoner who personally experienced the healing potential of reflexology whilst living in Canada, became a tutor for Dwight C Byers in the US. He later worked as a pioneer to establish another sector of the practitioner base in the UK, between the years 1970 and 1982, before returning to the US. During those formative years the 'road show' training technique was the fastest way of spreading awareness of reflexology techniques to all parts of the country. Charismatic practitioners like Dallamore held seminars and workshops with as many as 60 people in hired hotel rooms. Typically these early pioneers used enthusiastic attendees of previous sessions to help in what way they could. This type of short apprenticeship training has been heavily criticized, with demands for improved training and standardization of curricula primarily to protect the consumer from charlatans and poor practice (British Medical Association (BMA) 1986, 1993, Foundation for Integrated Medicine (FIM) 1997, House of Lords 2000). It is a tribute to the integrity of many reflexologists trained in this way that they found ways of developing and sustaining their practice in a professional manner.

During 1958, in Southern Germany, Hanne Marquardt, who originally trained in the UK as a nurse, was introduced to Eunice Ingham's work after completing therapeutic massage training. For 9 years she 'undertook a serious study' of Fitzgerald's Zone Theory (Lett 2000 p 14) before meeting Ingham, the still 'lively lady [aged 80 years]' (Marquardt 2000 p 3). Following this experience, Marquardt decided to develop her training only with healthcare professionals. Marquardt claimed to have developed further Fitzgerald's ideas, calling her method Reflex Zone Therapy of the feet (RZT). By 1980 the German training decentralized and other European centres for RZT training were opened including the UK. Ann Lett trained with Marquardt in 1980 and later became the first Principal of the British School of Reflex Zone Therapy for the Feet. This has relevance to this text in that RZT training was open only to healthcare practitioners. Clive O'Hara, who originally trained with Robert Dallamore, began a working partnership with the University of Manchester in 1991 to establish level 2 and 3 modules validated with both the University and the then English National Board for Nursing and Midwifery. This was the first course of its kind in the UK (Faltermeyer 1995). The success of this level of training can be measured by the publication of journal papers, the staging of a continuing series of national and international conferences for clinical reflexology and the production of this book. Now that we have traced the development of the early British reflexology training into education, it is appropriate to consider the current providers of reflexology programmes.

REFLEXOLOGY PROGRAMMES IN THE UK: DIFFERENT LEVELS OF PROVISION

For the purpose of reviewing the current provision these have been divided into three main groups of providers who offer different forms or bands of training and education. It is important to recognize that individual courses in those bands may produce practitioners with higher or even lower skills than claimed. It is also important to recognize that many students will also supplement their original preparation with postgraduate courses and supervision, enabling them to develop a higher level of skill.

COLLEGES OF FURTHER EDUCATION

A large number of therapists are trained at colleges of further education, usually in the hairdressing and beauty therapy departments (although an increasing number of colleges now include 'complementary therapies' in the department title). Some courses are introductory and non-vocational (without a qualification) and the rest are vocational using awarding bodies such as VTCT, ITEC and HNC/D. Some have used the designation 'salon reflexology' for this level or band, as it was felt that 'beauty level' sounded disparaging to the high level of skill that is attained by many beauty therapists. However, even the term 'salon' has been taken as downgrading and the Health and Beauty profession is currently searching for a term with which it will be content. Although awarded a 'diploma' or 'certificate' assuring competency, graduates often report a lack of confidence to then treat members of the public, even though they have been supervised and assessed working with clients. Many candidates learning reflexology by this route study other disciplines at the same time – massage, aromatherapy, Reiki, nutrition, counselling along with business skills. The diploma awarded following completion of these courses is often not equitable to the 'academic' diploma (level 2 – that is, year 2 of a university undergraduate programme) and is more likely to be in line with academic certificate level 1. College courses are funded by the Further Education Funding Council (FEFC) and often work with large class sizes, sometimes exceeding 20 students. Course duration can also vary from 20 (10 session × 2) hours to 108 (36 × 3) hours. An attractive feature is that these courses are usually part-time and often take place in the evening. These factors contribute to student fees being significantly less than in the private and university sectors. The cheaper cost is no doubt a reason that many health professionals attend these courses. Given that reflexology is an emerging and expanding profession, the teaching and mentoring may well vary from college to college. Anecdotal reports of novice reflexologists being hired to teach reflexology to groups with mixed ability and experience suggest that these institutions need to seek guidance from reflexology organizations not only to approve their programmes but also to formulate criteria for recruiting teachers of reflexology.

THE PRIVATE SECTOR

Private training schools and colleges offer a wide range of courses in reflexology. Many of these will have been started by reflexologists of many years experience, who will originate from, or be influenced by, different reflexology 'pioneers', as discussed in Section 1. Thus the reflexology techniques and underlying philosophy differ according to the background of the school, and training standards again differ. Some of these schools are in the beauty therapy sector, as described above, and could be said to teach 'salon reflexology' but would probably consider themselves offering 'practitioner level courses', whereas others fit into the category of 'clinical' reflexology. There are also 'road show' training arrangements in existence, which use hired hotel or university accommodation for a 1/2-day session teaching event each month for 4–6 sessions. Anecdotally, students often report feeling motivated to engage in reflexology practice by such exposure to dynamic and experienced teachers and practitioners of reflexology. This may be tempered by a lack of support and supervision locally to make the shift from competent to confident practitioner. Some private schools may not be formally linked with one of the national reflexology organizations, but such factors as their local reputation, postgraduate support and accessibility may be crucial in attracting students.

It is important to recognize that many practitioner programmes from the private and FE sectors incorporate assessment set at a level that may be in line with academic (university) level 1 and 2 with the relevant analysis of the subject built into the curriculum. These courses commonly follow the guidelines of a duration of 1 academic year; 200 minimum contact hours; minimum $2 \times 6 \times 6$ case study treatments; continuous practical assessment and either a written final assessment or minimum word assignment. These schools may also utilize an external examiner who will monitor the assessment process. This could include observing clinical assessments and/or moderating written assignments and examination papers. It is also important to recognize that some of the regulating bodies set national examination papers, take part in clinical assessments of students and review work of the schools and their teachers.

UNIVERSITY AND HIGHER EDUCATION

Academic level 3 (degree level) courses are in existence but not widely available. The Centre for Clinical Reflexology module was the basis from which the Manchester University level 3 module was written. This was the first one to be validated and run in the UK. There are one or two other reflexology modules at this level run by other universities but level 3 courses are rare. These programmes have an important role to play not only in helping students with their academic abilities, but also in raising the merit of reflexology as a valuable and attractive inclusion in graduate programmes. Significantly, graduates of the longest running programme have published in international peer-reviewed journals on the topic of reflexology (Dryden et al 1999, Mackereth 1999, Tipping and Mackereth 2000). There are degree programmes available in complementary medicine, but these do not usually include a practitioner qualification; graduates will have to complete a course recognized by a registered body in order to practise. This situation compartmentalizes the practice from the theory of complementary health care. For example, in the vocational sector, case studies are a common form of assessment and, while students may refer to zones, anatomy and physiology, and hygiene, it is unlikely that they would be expected critically to examine research evidence, ethical issues and therapeutic models. Box 2.1 gives examples of learning outcomes that may be ascribed to different scholarly levels.

Universities and higher education institutions are required to provide library and interlibrary loan facilities so that students have access to the available literature. Many private schools simply do not have these kinds of resources. Academic institutions are also subject to regular reviews of their teaching and research activities by internal and external panels of assessors. Again, not all reflexology schools have this level of monitoring. Internal markers and moderators as well as external examiners also assess students' work. The latter will attend examination boards and are required to produce an annual report. Many of these elements contribute to rigor in both managing and providing courses. These are also hurdles to jump over when establishing new programmes in established institutions. However, the popularity of complementary therapies amongst the general public has helped to raise the profile of reflexology and, increasingly, healthcare professionals are asking for courses that equip them to offer these kinds of interventions in healthcare settings. Universities and HE institutions need to attract students and as we enter the new millennium this is reflected in their interest in researching and teaching complementary therapies. It is important for healthcare professionals wishing to undertake reflexology training and education to examine carefully what courses offer in terms of registration and level of practice. If students want to work within healthcare environments they will need to discuss the choice of training with a clinical manager. Having a checklist is important in choosing the right

---

Box 2.1 Examples of learning outcome at different levels

- Level 1 (college certificate) – identify and describe the different theories of reflexology
- Level 2 (university diploma) – discuss the different theories of reflexology utilizing the available literature
- Level 3 (university degree) – critically review the theoretical basis of reflexology, exploring the wider literature and relevant research work on mechanisms of action

---

Box 2.2 Checklist for choosing a reflexology course

- Teacher(s) qualifications and experience
- Assessment strategy and academic level
- Approval and validating bodies, such as universities, colleges and professional reflexology organizations
- Educational resources, such as library facilities, internet access, teaching environment
- Quality of teaching packages, handouts and training manuals
- Access to clinical placements and practice clients
- Amount of supervision and tutorial support

reflexology programme (Box 2.2). It may also be useful to talk to other graduates from the course and seek advice from reflexology organizations.

THE NEED FOR REGULATION

In the 1990s there were several important milestones in the review and rec-ommendations for the education and regulation of complementary ther-apies, both in the UK and internationally. It is very likely that preparatory courses and requirements for registration and insurance will change dra-matically in the first decade of the twenty-first century. There are various factors influencing these developments. Healthcare professionals have been critical about the efficacy of complementary therapies and have called for improvements in the regulation and training of complementary practi-tioners (BMA 1986, 1993, FIM 1997, House of Lords 2000). Consumers and providers of complementary therapies require competent and accountable practitioners. Potential practitioners are themselves looking for the best course to suit their budget, time availability and educational and practice requirements. Lead bodies for the profession are also extremely active in developing to advance the standing of reflexology and to reassure and pro-tect the public and health professions. Budd & Mills (2000) believe that, given the variety of therapies, the way forward for individual therapy pro-fessions is self-regulation rather than statutory control. They have outlined the key activities that are necessary to assuring the public (Box 2.3).

THE WORK OF FIM AND THE REFLEXOLOGY FORUM

The Foundation for Integrated Medicine (FIM) was formed in 1996, with Prince Charles as president, and has become a key organization in leading the way in four identified key areas: complementary medicine research, education, regulation and provision (FIM 1997). A finding of the group was the need for both professional regulation of training and of practice. FIM

Box 2.3 Voluntary self-regulation activities Budd & Mills (2000)

- Maintains a register of individual members or member organizations
- Sets educational standards and an independent accreditation system for training establishments
- Maintains professional competence amongst its members with an adequate programme of continuing development
- Provides codes of conduct, ethics and practice
- Has in place a complaints procedure that is accessible to the public
- Requires members to have adequate professional indemnity insurance
- Has the capacity to represent the whole profession
- Includes external representation on executive councils to represent patients or clients and the wider public interest

---

Box 2.4   Recommended curriculum content (FIM 1997 p 22)

- Basic anatomy, physiology and pathology
- Fundamentals of orthodox medical diagnosis and guidelines for patient referral
- Complementary and alternative therapies and their potential uses, including the principles of diagnosis and practice
- Holistic models of health care
- Professional ethics
- The therapeutic relationship
- Impact of social, cultural, economic, employment and environmental factors on health
- Counselling skills
- Principles of quality management and audit
- Organizational skills, including record keeping
- Technical skills: ranging from prevention of cross-infection to information management (including data security to protect the privacy of medical records; use of information technology to access information; research and current best practice)

---

has been instrumental in supporting and encouraging the various disparate groups to come together to explore the possibility of one regulating body or council for each therapy and a standardized curriculum (Box 2.4).

Over the decades, many complementary therapy schools have sought to form associations and organizations to support their practitioners. Some of these groups have merged and, more recently, these associations have been exploring the establishment of one reflexology body, but this has not been without difficulties. Each organization has, over time, developed its own identity and approach, and the creation of one umbrella organization has led to much debate as to how to move forward and at the same time represent the interests of the individual associations. These associations have also been mindful that change might be forced upon the profession if they are not more proactive. The government has established Healthwork UK (the healthcare national training organization) and the Qualification and Curriculum Agency (QCA), reinforcing the need to work together to develop one voice for reflexology (Duncan 2000). This is essential if the profession wishes to communicate effectively with the public, providers of complementary therapies, healthcare professionals and government bodies.

In line with the 'lead body' proposal put forward by the FIM (1997) a working party was set up from the various reflexology organizations. This 'lead body' was intended to represent a minimum of 80% of qualified and practising reflexologists. The aim was to devise a way for each reflexology group, no matter what size, to have an equal and fair representation and, as Duncan (2000 p 7) states 'with this strong constitutional platform in place the Reflexology Forum was born'.

The most important first step for the Reflexology Forum is the development of the National Occupational Standards and a national framework of qualifications. The National Occupational Standards provide the Forum with a structure from which to develop a qualification framework and the

---

Box 2.5 The aims of the Reflexology Forum (cited in Mills & Budd 2000 p 78)

- Represent the majority of qualified reflexologists in the country
- Maintain the independence and diversity of member organizations
- Work for the benefit of reflexology
- Develop National Occupational Standards and a national framework of qualifications
- Work in consultation with Healthwork UK and the Quality and Curriculum Agency
- Promote research into reflexology
- Encourage professional development of reflexology
- Be governed by a set of standards for self-regulation
- Maintain and develop good working practices with a view to safeguarding the general public
- Explore and discuss the future possible developments of the Reflexology Forum to include discussions regarding the setting up of a General Reflexology Council

---

appropriate regulatory system for reflexology. The last of the aims listed for the Reflexology Forum (Box 2.5) includes such developments as forming a General Reflexology Council (GRC). This would require the disbanding of all current reflexology organizations, to be replaced by the GRC; this is currently being explored and may take time to achieve. Although it is important to establish a standard for a common foundation programme for all reflexologists, it is important to recognize that education does not cease once qualified. Most of the reflexology organizations evolved not only to register and arrange insurance, but also to support and help members to develop their practice.

CONTINUING EDUCATION FOR REFLEXOLOGISTS

Continuing education is judged to be a necessary process to ensure safe and ever-improving practice and a hallmark of professional self-regulation (Budd & Mills 2000). There are, of course, many ways to do this (Box 2.6), but perhaps the most important factor is an individual's motivation for the activity. Time and financial costs, as well as availability of suitable means of ongoing education, cannot be ignored. Some organizations recommend that their members commit themselves to a minimum requirement of, for example, 10 hours a year. This will usually need to be evidenced by copies of attendance certificates, verification of supervisory contact by a supervisor or a written report by the practitioner of their continuing education activities.

The Centre for Health Research and Evaluation (CHRE), at the University of Greenwich, commissioned by the Department of Health, has provided a framework for continuing professional development for complementary and alternative medicine (CHRE 2000). This involved a major national research project with 30 universities, 17 royal colleges and professional organizations and 35 complementary and alternative medicine training establishments. Reflective practice was one of many strategies proposed in the framework for safeguarding and improving clinical practice (Box 2.6). The process of reflective practice has been defined as 'reviewing an experience of practice in order to describe, analyse and evaluate and so inform learning from practice' (Reid 1993 p 305). This can be done *in* or *on* practice, requiring careful consideration of interactions, situations and interventions, at the time or shortly after the event. Models of reflection typically suggest practitioners examine key components of an experience, which can include ethical, practical and safety concerns, personal meaning, existing knowledge, sources of further information, and alternative strategies and their possible outcomes (Gibbs 1988, Johns 1994).

ENGAGING IN REFLECTIVE PRACTICE AND SUPERVISION

Opportunities for reflexology-specific support and guidance were found to be scarce for individual practitioners working on their own in a ward, hospital or community clinic, or in private practice (CHRE 2000). If time and space can be provided for supervision meetings, the practitioner can be helped to take the process of reflection into everyday practice. Reflective practice and supervision have been identified as a means of exploring the therapeutic role of the practitioner (Jones 1995). For nurses and midwives, supervision has been identified as an important part of supporting and safeguarding an individual practitioner's scope of professional practice (UKCC 1995). From a legal perspective it has been suggested (Tingle 1995) that clinical supervision could operate as a clinical risk management

---

Box 2.6   Examples of continuing education activities

- Reflective practice, incorporating a structured review of clinical skills, events, professional interactions, and ongoing and potential learning activities
- Clinical supervision – contracted monthly individual or group sessions facilitated by an experienced practitioner
- Mentoring/preceptorship – regular supervisory contact with an experienced practitioner for the first year post-qualification
- Educational events – attendance at national and international conferences, study days and workshops
- Journal club – each member reports back on an article/chapter/educational event
- Clinical supervision – meeting monthly with a supervisor either individually or in a group
- Peer support group – informal 1–2-monthly meetings to exchange treatments and share practice issues
- Networking and communicating regularly with colleagues by post, telephone, e-mail and readers' letter pages of journals and newsletters
- Accessing information via the Internet, libraries and associations' newsletters and journals

---

Box 2.7 Clinical supervision contract (Mackereth 2000)

Shared responsibilities for:

- agreeing the venue, dates and times for supervision
- avoiding rescheduling sessions where possible (ideally 24-hour notice)
- the maintenance of confidentiality within limits*
- regularly reviewing the usefulness of the supervision
- giving 2 sessions notice if discontinuing/changing supervision arrangements
- negotiating and clarifying the focus of the supervision work at each session

* Limits of confidentiality include acts/intentions that are illegal, breaks the participants' code of conduct or infringes their employment-related disciplinary policies

---

tool that could help to reduce complaints and even litigation. Seeking and organizing supervision, in discussion with a line or clinic manager, can help to reassure patients and colleagues that accountability and quality enhancement will be paramount to the provision of reflexology.

The activity of clinical supervision was first described in the work of psychotherapists and was later incorporated into counselling practice; more recently, nurses and midwives have been engaging in the process (Butterworth & Faugier 1995). Mackereth (1997) suggests that nurses using complementary therapies can be supported to become more 'potent' in their therapeutic work by engaging regularly in supervision. In a project providing reflexology on a hospital ward Johns' (1994) trigger questions for reflection and monthly clinical supervision meetings were reported as providing insight and valued support for the practitioners (Cromwell et al 1999). Typically, supervision involves meeting on a regular basis with a facilitator, this can be as an individual or in a small group. Essential to the process and the relationship is the establishment of a working contract (Box 2.7). Hope-Spencer (2000), a teacher and reflexology practitioner, argues from her own experience of working in medical settings that supervision should be considered an 'important adjunct to offering support to the student and practitioner' (p 21).

TEACHING AND SUPPORTING STUDENTS IN HEALTH CARE SETTINGS

As with any practical skill, becoming a good teacher of reflexology includes achieving, maintaining and developing teaching and clinical expertise. With complementary therapies this mix can be a problem as many practitioners learn their skill as mature students (Rankin-Box 1997) so the time available to qualify and develop as both practitioners and teachers is reduced. With greater integration within the health service there is an added problem in that nurses and midwives who expand into complementary practices may have less time to devote to a therapy, given that a complete treatment of clinical reflexology usually lasts for an hour. It was suggested by the work of Dryden et al (1999) that treatments could be adapted by health professionals, equipped with reflexology skills, to suit a shorter time frame and with positive therapeutic outcomes for patients. Intervening with reflexology in clinical situations requires specific skills and knowledge and not all reflexology courses can prepare students to work in healthcare settings. This will require additional training programmes facilitated by experienced practitioners. Many of the contributors to this book facilitate short courses and provide supervision to reflexologists wishing to develop in specialist areas such as palliative and maternity care. Figure 2.1 shows the author supervising a clinical reflexology student – a midwife – who is intending to develop a reflexology service in a maternity care unit. Participation in these learning activities also assures providers and recipients of reflexology that their practitioners are developing and maintaining practice.

The shortage of speciality teachers in complementary therapies and health care has been recognized by Nicholl (1995). One option could be to recruit practitioners from outside the health service to contribute towards educational programmes, but they may lack teaching skills or be unfamiliar with healthcare issues. This could be overcome by team teaching, for example, two facilitators, each with different skills and clinical experience to offer, contributing to classroom and tutorial activities (Faltermeyer 1995). When two or more teachers have input into the programme there is a need to share and

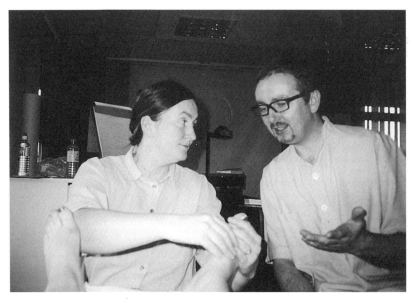

Figure 2.1   Clinical practice being supervised. Mackereth P. reproduced from Journal of Complementary Therapies in Nursing and Midwifery 1999; 5(3):68

speak the same language so as not to confuse students. Although confusion is good at challenging what we do not know and therefore need to find out, it can undermine a student's confidence, particularly at foundation level. These problems can be resolved by careful preparation and evaluation of teaching strategies by both the teachers and the students.

As clinical reflexology courses develop there is a need to support students and teachers. This must start in the planning stage, taking into account educational resources and identifying potential mentors for students in clinical practice and teachers networking locally and nationally (Faltermeyer 1995). This provides opportunities to share developing expertise in a specific clinical area. For example, in maternity care, links can be made with practitioners through the Complementary Maternity Forum (see Useful addresses, p. 32). Sharing resources and experience is another important reason for graduates and teachers to be active in reflexology associations (Nicholl 1995). Many associations offer student membership and reductions in conference and workshops fees in order to encourage continuing professional education and networking.

CONCLUSION

This chapter has reviewed the past, current and future developments in the preparation of reflexologists, and has looked at regulation issues and continuing education activities. It is important for both students and teachers

---

Box 2.8 Key recommendations in developing clinical reflexology

- One national regulating body with networking internationally
- Teachers who have both educational and reflexology qualifications
- Reflexologists working in healthcare settings contributing to teaching and supervision
- Educational partnerships between practitioners working in private and public complementary therapy services
- Incorporate skills in reflective practice in all reflexology programmes
- Increased provision of clinical courses approved and monitored by higher education institutions and regulatory bodies
- Requirement for all reflexologists to engage in and provide evidence of professional development
- Increased body of quality literature, including critical examination of reflexology theory, practice and research
- Opportunities for reflexologists to network (local, national and international conferences and workshops)
- Development of specialist reflexology courses and means of supervision
- Greater provision of reflexology within healthcare practice
- Increased disseminating of information about reflexology to the public, healthcare professionals and reflexologists (e.g. worldwide web and the use of the media, literature, etc.)

to acknowledge that the profession is growing rapidly at a time of technology advance and consumer interest in the benefits of reflexology. It is also important to examine critically how the profession might best organize itself to provide quality education and the promotion of continuing education. This chapter has discussed the key issues and challenges related to education and its regulation, highlighting the work of the pioneers and leaders of reflexology, the Reflexology Forum and the Foundation for Integrated Medicine. Box 2.8 summarizes some of the key recommendations for the immediate and future development of the profession.

REFERENCES

Adamson S, Harris E, Kerr S. The reflexology partnership. London: Kyle Cathie; 1995.
British Medical Association (BMA). Alternative therapy. Report of the Board of Science and Education. London: British Medical Association; 1986.
British Medical Association (BMA). Complementary medicine. New approaches to good practice. Oxford: British Medical Association/Oxford University Press; 1993.
Budd S, Mills S. Regulatory prospects for complementary and alternative medicine: information pack. Exeter: Centre for Complementary Health Studies, University of Exeter on behalf of the Department of Health; 2000.
Butterworth T, Faugier J. Clinical supervision in nursing, midwifery and health visiting: developments, contracts and monitoring. A 2nd briefing paper. Manchester: School of Nursing Studies, University of Manchester; 1995.
Cant SL, Sharma U. Professionalization of complementary medicine in the United Kingdom. Complementary Therapies in medicine 1996; 4:157–162.
Centre for Health Research and Evaluation (CHRE). Continuing professional development for complementary and alternative medicine. London: CHRE/the University of Greenwich School of Health; 2000.
Cromwell C, Dryden SL, Jones D, Mackereth PA. 'Just the ticket': case studies, reflections and clinical supervision (part III) Complementary Therapies in Nursing and Midwifery 1999; 5(2):42–45.
Dougans I. The complete illustrated guide to reflexology. Dorset: Element Books; 1996.
Dryden SL, Holden SD, Mackereth P. 'Just the ticket': integrating massage and reflexology in practice (part I). Complementary Therapies in Nursing and Midwifery 1998; 4(6):154–159.
Dryden SL, Holden SD, Mackereth P. 'Just the ticket': the findings of a pilot complementary therapy service (part II) Complementary Therapies in Nursing and Midwifery 1999; 5(1):15–18.
Duncan S. The reflexology forum. Reflexions. Journal of the Association of Reflexologists 2000; 58:6–7.
Faltermeyer TS. Working towards quality – developing an approved course. Complementary Therapies in Nursing and Midwifery 1995; 1(5):138–142.
Foundation for Integrated Medicine (FIM). Integrated Healthcare: a way forward for the next five years? London: FIM; 1997.
Gibbs G. Learning by doing: a guide to teaching and learning methods. Oxford: Further Education Unit, Oxford Polytechnic (now Oxford Brookes University); 1988.
Gore A. Reflexology. London: Optima; 1990.
Hall N. Reflexology – a step by step guide. Dorset: Element Books; 1997.
Hope-Spencer J. The case for supervision Reflexions. Journal of the Association of Reflexologists. 2000; 58:21–23.
House of Lords. Select Committee on Science and Technology, Complementary and alternative medicine, HL Paper 123. London: House of Lords; 2000.
Johns C. Nuances of reflection. Journal of Clinical Nursing 1994; 3(2):71–75.

Jones A. Taking counsel. Nursing Times 1995; 91(26):28–29.

Lett A. Reflex zone therapy for health professionals. London: Churchill Livingstone; 2000.

Mackereth PA. Clinical supervision for 'potent' practice. Complementary Therapies in Nursing and Midwifery 1997; 3:38–41.

Mackereth P. An introduction to catharsis and the healing crisis in reflexology. Complementary Therapies in Nursing and Midwifery 1999; 5(3):67–74.

Mackereth P. Clinical supervision and complementary therapies In: Rankin-Box D, ed. Nurses' handbook of complementary therapies. London: Churchill Livingstone; 2000.

Marquardt H. Reflexotherapy for the feet. New York: Thieme; 2000.

Mills S, Budd S. Professional organisation of complementary and alternative medicine in the United Kingdom 2000. Exeter: Centre for the Complementary Health Studies. University of Exeter; 2000.

Nicholl LK. Complementary therapies in nurse education – the need for specialist teachers. Complementary Therapies in Nursing and Midwifery 1995; 1(3):69–72.

Norman L. The reflexology handbook. London: Piatkus; 1988.

Rankin-Box D. Therapies in practice: a survey assessing nurses' use of complementary therapies. Complementary Therapies in Nursing and Midwifery 1997; 3(4):92–99.

Reid B. But we're doing it already! Exploring a response to the concept of reflective practice in order to improve its facilitation. Nurse Education Today 1993; 13:305–309.

Tingle J. Clinical supervision is an effective risk management tool. British Journal of Nursing 1995; 4(14):794–795.

Tipping E, Mackereth P. A concept analysis: the effect of reflexology on homeostasis to establish and maintain lactation. Complementary Therapies in Nursing and Midwifery 2000; 6(4):189–198.

Tiran D. The use of complementary therapies in midwifery practice a focus on reflexology. Complementary Therapies in Nursing and Midwifery 1996; 2(2):32–37.

UKCC. Position statement on clinical supervision for nursing and health visiting. London: United Kingdom Central Council for Nursing, Midwifery and Health Visiting; 1995.

USEFUL CONTACTS

The Foundation for Integrated Medicine
12 Chillingworth Road, London, N7 8QJ
Tel: 0207 688 1881
E-mail: enquiries@fimed.org
Website: http://www.fimed.org.uk

Reflexology Forum
208 Croham Valley Road, South Croydon, Surrey, CR 7RB
Tel: 0208 6510582
E-mail: Jandec44@aol.com

Complementary Maternity Forum
c/o Denise Tiran, Principal Lecturer, School of Health, The University of Greenwich,
Avery Hill University Campus, Mansion Site, Bexley Road, Eltham, London
Tel: 0208 331 8494
Fax: 0208 331 9926
E-mail: M. D.Tiran@gre.ac.uk

Royal College of Nursing Complementary Therapies in Nursing Forum
Royal College of Nursing, 20 Cavendish Square, London, WIG 0RN
Tel: 0345 726 100

3

Challenging the 'rules' of reflexology

Clive S O'Hara

Abstract

Modern reflexology is still comparatively young and continuing to develop so there
are few authoritative clinicians in the field who are able to make definitive guidelines
for practice. However, many early reflexology textbooks have taken a cautious
approach to the treatment of clients and the position of the practitioner in relation to
colleagues in conventional health care. This has led to certain 'rules' which appear to
have become absolute in many schools of reflexology: do not diagnose; do not
prescribe; do not treat specific illnesses; do not treat pregnant women (Kunz & Kunz
1984, Norman 1995). However, reflexology is now used to a much greater extent
within conventional health care, both by those already working in the National Health
Service, such as nurses, midwives and physiotherapists, and by independent
practitioners contracted into the health services. This provides increasing opportunity
to demonstrate evidence of the efficacy, safety and benefits of reflexology in a variety
of clinical settings, although such evidence may require an adjustment of previously
held views, particularly amongst conventional healthcare professionals. With the
encouragement of the Foundation for Integrated Medicine (FIM 1997) and the
development of the Reflexology Forum (Mills & Budd 2000) greater integration is
becoming increasingly possible. This chapter debates and challenges the 'rules' for
practice and considers how a more flexible approach may be beneficial for health
care in general and facilitate the incorporation of reflexology as a viable therapeutic
intervention within conventional health care.

Key words: diagnosis, prescribing, contraindications, stimulation,
normalization, homeostasis/homeodynamics, solar plexus/coeliac
ganglion

It is impossible to consider the use of reflexology without recognizing that
the standards of education, training and levels of experience of practitioners
have improved dramatically in recent years, in line with the government's
general strategy for expanding the availability to the public, acceptance by
the medical professions and the credibility of many complementary therapies (House of Lords 2000). Once qualified, reflexologists progress through
the stages from 'novice' to 'competent' to 'expert' (Benner 1984) but practitioners at any level must first assess a client, interpret their findings and

---

Box 3.1 The 'Reflexology Package'

Feature	Benefit
• Substantial treatment duration	Quality personal time for client
• One-to-one situation	Potential for communication
• Face-to-face – constant eye contact	Encourages communication
• Tactile – continuous physical contact	Employs therapeutic touch – but . . .
• Preserves personal space	. . . doesn't invade personal space boundary
• Non-invasive technique	No equipment or pharmacological substances
• Can provide diagnostic information	In addition to being a therapeutic treatment

---

then decide upon the type and appropriateness of intended treatment (Lett 2000), declining to treat anyone whose condition is outside the limitations of their personal practice, training and experience.

However, as individual practitioners gain more experience, competence and confidence in their abilities, some may stretch the boundaries of practice and move beyond those 'absolutes' about which they learned as a student reflexologist. This process occurs in many professions – take, for example, the efforts of surgeons such as the late Christian Barnard, who performed the first heart transplant. Without a certain amount of experimentation, no progress would be made and a profession would not move forwards. On the other hand, it is essential that any deviation from standard practice is undertaken only after consolidation of basic knowledge and skills, plus further and continuing education in order to understand fully the implications of the intended developments.

It is also important to recognize the aims and outcomes of reflexology treatment and the effects that it may have upon an individual. Kunz & Kunz (1984) suggest that reflexology increases the sense of relaxation and wellbeing, improves cardiovascular, lymphatic and neurological function, and restores and maintains homeostasis. If these effects are combined with the features of the therapeutic intervention (see Chapter 7), a 'reflexology package' can be identified, which has several benefits for the client (Box 3.1). Ethically and legally, the reflexologist should 'do no harm' to the client and this forms the basis for practice when considering any adaptations to their personal practice, including the introduction of new techniques or contravening guidelines which formed part of their original training.

THE 'RULES' OF REFLEXOLOGY

The 'rules' included in the training of reflexologists are intended as a means of protecting both clients and practitioners. Some guidelines are included at pre-registration training level because further knowledge, understanding and experience is required before treating a specific client group, such as women in the first trimester of pregnancy (see Chapter 10). Others are based on differences in legal definitions and the current regulatory status of reflexologists in relation to conventional healthcare practitioners. Greater integration of complementary therapies into orthodox healthcare has resulted in in-depth explorations of basic and post-basic training, regulation, insurance and other issues, which are gradually producing highly competent and knowledgeable practitioners, able to take their place with credibility and professionalism in the wider healthcare arena. Let us, then, explore further some of these 'rules' that have previously placed somewhat unnecessary restrictions on practice.

'REFLEXOLOGISTS SHOULD NOT DIAGNOSE'

The issue of whether or not reflexologists should diagnose fuels much debate and reflexologists are not the only group that holds strong opinions. The situation is compounded by the legal status of reflexologists in the UK, for English Common Law continues to permit independent practice and there is no legal definition of what constitutes 'diagnosis'. This is in direct contradiction to the Napoleonic Law that applies to much of Europe, in which 'diagnoses' can be made only by medically qualified practitioners. In addition, because modern reflexology started in the US, many guidelines for practice are written with American legislation in mind, where strict licensing exists and policies appear to be dictated by the threat of litigation.

Currently in the UK, two umbrella complementary organizations take opposing views. The Institute for Complementary Medicine (1994) states that practitioners may make a diagnosis within the terms of their own discipline and determine a programme of treatment whereas, in contrast, the British Complementary Medical Association has been associated with moves for increased deference to (orthodox) medical diagnosis and the policy that they will not attempt diagnoses where these can be provided by a doctor (Mills & Budd 2000).

The dictionary explains the term 'diagnosis' as coming from the Greek *dia* meaning 'through' and *gnosis* meaning 'knowledge', and defines it as 'the determination of the *nature of* a case of disease' (Dorland's Medical Dictionary 1994) or 'the thorough analysis of facts or problems in order to *gain understanding*' (Collins Modern English Dictionary 1987). The Dictionary of Medical Terms (1994) expands this by adding: 'determining the nature of a patient's disease or injury by consideration of signs and symptoms (elicited by examination and questioning), together with any test results, X-rays or scans, and a knowledge of the patient's history'. However, 'determining the nature of disease' does not necessarily mean attaching a specific title to a set of signs or symptoms but can apply in general terms and to part of the process that leads to a conclusion. It is not always possible for a single individual or discipline to reach a conclusion in isolation and a team approach may be needed to document the data and reach a diagnosis. There are also different categories of diagnosis. Dorland's Medical Dictionary (1994) lists 16 such as 'clinical diagnosis – diagnosis based on signs, symptoms and laboratory tests during life'. This list could be expanded to include allopathic diagnosis, complementary medical diagnosis and reflexology diagnosis.

It is interesting to note a difference in attitude to reflexology diagnosis between different texts. Kaye & Matchan (1978) suggest that *any* health advice borders on diagnosis and prescribing and state categorically that reflexologists should not diagnose, prescribe, promise to cure or help a specific problem, although they admit that these rules may be restrictive and unreasonable. Conversely, Gooseman-Legger (1986) believes that reflexology can be an important *addition* to differential diagnosis and Gore (1990) feels that 'one of reflexology's greatest and most impressive strengths is its ability to make accurate diagnoses of conditions and symptoms'. Many reflexology authorities remain cautious about the right of practitioners to make a diagnosis (Dougans 1996, Gillanders 1994, Kunz & Kunz 1984, Norman 1995) but assert that the therapy can be 'devastatingly accurate' in determining the state of a person's health (Kunz & Kunz 1984 p 75). Marquardt (2000 p 161) suggests that the therapeutic and diagnostic aspects of the therapy cannot easily be separated. Gillanders advocates reflexologists working alongside the medical profession but, somewhat worryingly, Norman (1995 p 96) feels that 'lay people can use reflexology to pinpoint or confirm diagnoses'. Wildwood (1994), an aromatherapist, uses reflexology to aid her diagnosis and selection of essential oils, but this mixing of therapies poses yet another area for debate, which is not dealt with here (Case study 3.1).

Case study 3.1 Reflexology as a diagnostic process – a limitation and contradiction

A 19-year-old beauty therapist decided to add to her three years of quality training at a college of further education by enrolling on an extra 22-week aromatherapy course. During this 3-hours-a-week syllabus there was one evening session dedicated to studying reflexology for diagnostic use. Upon completion of the course she received a diploma and obtained insurance to practise using essential oils, which she sometimes chose based on making a diagnosis of her clients' health problems by using reflexology. Enthused with the potency of this diagnostic tool she enrolled for a further 22-week vocational course in reflexology. At the end of this further training she was informed that although now she held a diploma in (salon) reflexology she was in no way permitted to diagnose and, further, her insurance did not permit her to treat any person with a medical condition unless she had written permission from the doctor. It is a contradiction that with 3 hours training, she could use reflexology to diagnose as an aromatherapist but after 66 more hours, she could not diagnose as a reflexologist.

Kunz & Kunz (1984) take the view that reflexology will work without diagnosis but this seems unprofessional in the current climate of litigation and the increasing dependence upon evidence-based medical practice. Whether or not the reflexologist decides to make a clinical diagnosis may depend on the aim of the session: however, although 'salon' reflexology is intended purely for relaxation and 'sports' reflexology is often used for pain relief, one would hope that certain fundamental health questions are asked in order to avoid inappropriate therapy.

It is the very potential of reflexology to locate specific reflex areas on the feet (or hands) directly related to distal areas of the body that may be affected pathologically that makes reflexology a useful diagnostic tool in clinical practice. It is important that the reflexologist has sufficient knowledge to interpret correctly the signs from the feet and the symptoms reported by the client to assist in making a diagnosis from which a decision regarding appropriate treatment can be made.

What makes 'diagnosis' difficult for newly qualified or inexperienced reflexologists is often a lack of full understanding of the implications of changes in a specific reflex zone, especially whether the changes represent physiological or pathological changes. This understanding may seem less imperative when a therapist agrees to treat a referral from a doctor or GP who has already decided that the patient's condition warrants reflexology treatment. However, the fact that many GPs do not yet have sufficient awareness of reflexology to be able to refer with authority highlights the need for reflexologists to be trained to make these decisions for themselves. In fact, it would be unfair to ask for approval of a GP if s/he is not familiar with reflexology, its potential benefits, limitations and contraindications. This is partly due to the fact that reflexology is not yet spread widely through the conventional health services, but increasing incorporation of the therapy into mainstream care should help to make medical staff more aware.

A reflexologist and a GP have different levels of responsibility. The GP carries a caseload of patients who generally consult only when their health status changes, whereas reflexology clients have, at present, usually chosen specifically to receive the therapy. However, until all doctors and GPs have sufficient awareness of the extent and limitations of reflexology to be able to make an informed decision whether one of their patients should have treatment, the responsibility to proceed with reflexology should remain with the qualified, insured reflexologist (Case study 3.2). An important part of this qualification is the ability to identify any contraindications to treatment, which is essentially part of the diagnostic process.

Resistance to reflexology diagnosis amongst medical practitioners is understandable, because they would not wish ill-equipped lay persons to misinform and scare patients with allopathic 'labels' that they are not qualified to offer. The British Register of Complementary Practitioners' (1994)

Case study 3.2   Reflexology as a diagnostic tool – its extent and limitations

A female client presented with a marked increase in frequency of micturition, stating that she had a kidney infection. During the consultation no other symptoms of this infection were disclosed. During treatment, the reflex areas for the urinary system were not sensitive, but the pancreas reflexes were. Already the practitioner was silently considering the possibility of diabetes. The opportunity to talk during the hour-long treatment revealed the client's continual thirst. At the end of the session the practitioner told the client that her pancreas reflex was sensitive and suggested firmly that the client ask her GP for a blood test. This revealed that she needed treatment for diabetes, which was then administered by the doctor. She still, however, continued to visit the reflexologist regularly, which did not conflict with her medication because of the frequent self-monitoring of blood sugar levels and visits to the GP's diabetic clinic. Despite being a clinical reflexologist, this practitioner had no other medical training so did not feel qualified to label diabetes or administer any tests personally; a reflexologist–medic might have named the condition in allopathic terms and possibly tested blood or urine as extra information to pass to the client's GP.

Code of Practice and Ethics warns that 'no attempt should be made to describe a complementary diagnosis in allopathic terms unless the practitioner is so qualified'. Unfortunately, this does still happen occasionally, with reflexologists (and other complementary practitioners) overstepping the mark, either through lack of professional self-awareness or from professional arrogance (Case study 3.3).

It must be stressed that there is no claim that reflexology techniques alone can furnish a diagnosis, at least in allopathic terms. The British Register of Complementary Practitioners (1994) advocates care in describing symptoms when referring patients for allopathic diagnoses or tests but suggests that a reflexologist is qualified to make a medical diagnosis that might include sensitivity in certain areas, although it may be outside their competence to put an allopathic name to the condition. It is plain the term 'medical diagnosis' as used above refers to complementary medicine in that it is used in contrast to the term 'allopathic', which is used in its widest sense to refer to conventional or orthodox medicine.

However, before reflexology diagnoses can be consistent the charts that map the reflex points must be standardized. For example, a condition affecting the pituitary gland cannot be reliably suggested if the reflex zone

---

Case study 3.3   A limitation – 'overstepping the mark' with a 'diagnosis'

A 45-year-old woman who referred to herself as a healer enrolled on a short vocational reflexology course at night school with the intention of gaining some qualification to legitimize her healing activity. Using a foot chart during her hands-on treatment practice, she not only told a client that there was 'a lumpy part on the pituitary gland' but also said that the heart was 'very tender'. The client went home worried about brain tumours and heart attacks and was not only distraught but then informed her GP of the 'reflexologist's diagnosis'. The doctor's opinion of reflexology did not help him warm towards the concept of integrated medicine.

for the pituitary gland differs from one practitioner's chart to another. Ingham (1984) originally placed the pituitary gland zone in the centre of the plantar hallux. This is not consistent with the zone arrangement, for the pituitary gland is anatomically in the centre of the head, so the pituitary reflex point should be in zone 1 of the foot. Most other reflexologists agree that the pituitary reflex is the 'peak' of the big toe 'where the whorl of the toe print converges into a central point', which, although differing from one client's toe shape to another, is usually in zone 3 (Fig. 3.1; Fig. 3.2, Plate 1) (Dougans 1996). Ingham (1984) did not chart the area for the hypothalamus; the relationship between this part of the brain and the pituitary gland became better documented as the twentieth century progressed. Dougans (1996) and Norman (1995) both place the area for the hypothalamus in zone 1, which, by anatomical reasoning, must be in the identical area to that of the pituitary gland. Their size together is less than a zone width and the two are physiologically joined by tissue, nerve and blood supply to the extent that they are one. As they cannot be separated by reflexology identification, the logical conclusion must be that,

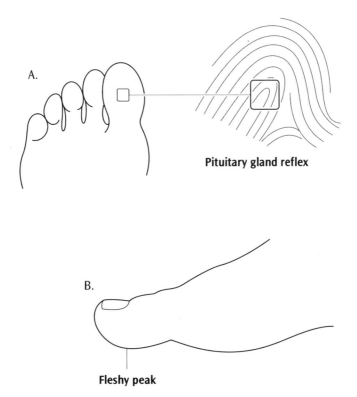

Pituitary gland reflex

Fleshy peak

Figure 3.1 Universally accepted location of the pituitary gland. A. Pituitary gland reflex. B. Medial/plantar view of the fleshy peak, showing the peak at the centre of the whorls.

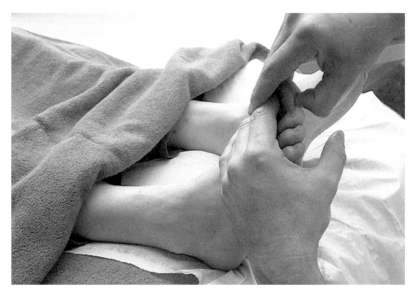

Figure 3.2   Practitioner working the pituitary area (see also Plate 1). Photo courtesy of Katie Spruce BA (Hons), medical photographer, Christie Hospital NHS Trust, with permission.

where the pituitary gland proves to be, the hypothalamus must be also. Interestingly, those charts that place the hypothalamus in a different zone to the pituitary gland also put the more recently mapped pineal gland in the same zone as the hypothalamus (Fig. 3.3) (Dougans 1996, Norman 1995). As any anatomy and physiology text will demonstrate (e.g. Solomon et al 1990) far less is known about the pineal gland than the pituitary and the hypothalamus and it is likely that Norman (1995) and Dougans (1996) based their judgements on theory rather than practice.

Other differences between charts can be seen in relation to the arm, elbow, leg and knee reflex areas (Fig. 3.4) (Lett 2000, Marquardt 2000, Norman 1995, Wagner 1987) and the oesophagus (Norman 1995, Wagner 1987). Probably the first reflex area with which most reflexologists become familiar at the beginning of their training is the solar plexus, more recently identified in modern anatomy texts as the coeliac ganglion or plexus (Lett 2000, Solomon et al 1990). It is surprising that the majority of new reflexologists do not notice that the location of this first learned reflex is not where it should be according to the zones. Clearly, there should be one solar/coeliac plexus in centre of the pair of feet in zone 1, whereas the majority unquestioningly accept its placement in zone 3 on the diaphragm lateral zone line on both feet – where it most definitely can be found, especially on stressed clients (Fig. 3.5) (compare Dougans 1996, Kunz & Kunz 1984, Norman 1995, Wagner 1987 with Lett 2000, Marquardt 2000). The fact that the dated term 'solar plexus' is harder to find in the more recently written human biology texts, where it is now referred to as the 'coeliac gan-

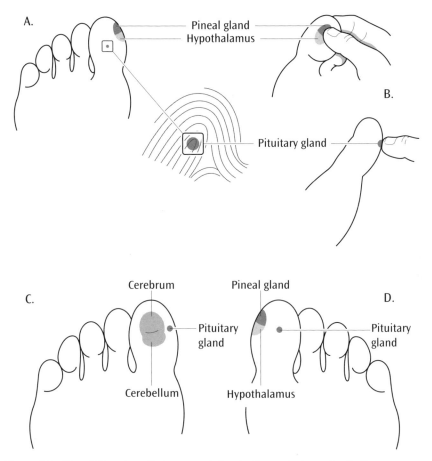

Figure 3.3 The pituitary, hypothalamus and pineal reflexes. A. According to Dougans (1996). B. According to Stormer (1992). C. According to Marquardt (2000). The hypothalamus and pineal gland are not mapped in this text. D. According to Norman (1995).

glion', coupled with the reality that this reflex location is not zonally correct, has led to the assertion that the solar plexus does not really exist (Arnold 2000). The naming and reflex location of the solar/coeliac plexus illustrates the need for clinical reflexologists continually to challenge the rigour of basic training and to recognize the importance of continuing professional development.

The reflexology foot charts included in the appendix at the end of this chapter (and as Plates 2, 3 and 4) illustrate the value of a challenging approach and continual professional development. The additional mapping of reflex points from the 'Foundation' chart of 1981 and 1991 to the 'Advanced' chart of 1996 includes pineal gland; hypothalamus; thymus; nose; teeth; duodenum; axillary, mammary and inguinal lymphatics, thoracic and lymphatic ducts; hepatic and splenic flexures; and the anus. Renaming

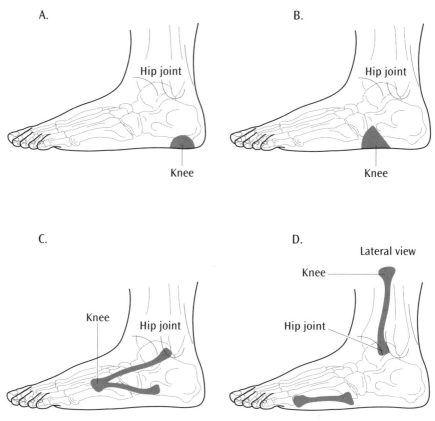

Figure 3.4 The knee reflex. A. According to Dougans (1996). B. According to Norman (1995). C. According to Stormer (1992). D. According to Lett (2000).

includes the term 'cardiac sphincter' to replace 'hiatus hernia' and the dropping of the term 'solar plexus', which is replaced by 'coeliac plexus'.

The imposing of the 'do not diagnose' rule has served a vital role in curbing the tendency of trainee and lay practitioners to attach allopathic disease labels to their clients when they are not qualified to do this. Many clients have hitherto mistakenly believed that diagnosis is the sole purpose of reflexology, although professional clinical reflexologists should decline to continue with a consultation if a client refuses to divulge prior history and symptoms purely in an attempt to challenge the reflexologist to identify their condition. When clients display such a motive the situation could be handled by referring them to the therapeutic contract (see Chapters 7 and 9). However, reflexology has progressed as a profession and, with this, the awareness of the public is improving, leading them to have greater understanding of the clinical nature of the therapy.

The majority of reflexologists will each have their own amazing accounts of the diagnostic power of reflexology, these experiences sometimes occur-

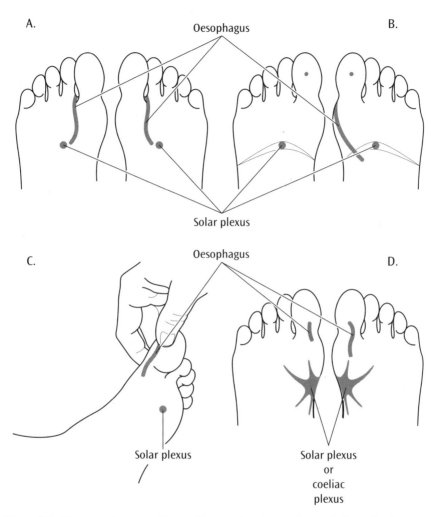

Figure 3.5 The oesophagus and the coeliac or solar plexus reflexes. A. According to Dougans (1996). B. According to Norman (1995). C. According to Stormer (1992). D. According to Lett (2000).

ring early in training. Although anecdotal proof is not scientifically valid in medical research, large quantities of frequently reoccurring evidence are hard to ignore. By its very nature, a reflexology chart is diagnostic in locating areas of the body linked to points on the feet and hands and inviting practitioners to identify which points have significance. If this element were to form no part of a reflexology session, a treatment pattern or sequence would be the only aid required – the chart would be irrelevant and become redundant. If, because of recent small-scale negative research, the diagnostic aspect of reflexology is to be dismissed (White et al 2000), medicine could be guilty of 'throwing the baby out with the bath water'. This would be especially ill timed if, as the integration theme of this text indicates, the opportunities and facilities to implement significant medical research and audit are now becoming available.

'REFLEXOLOGISTS SHOULD NOT PRESCRIBE'

Kunz & Kunz (1984 p 75) state that 'one of the greatest temptations in reflexology is to combine treatments with nutritional advice. The urge to diagnose is often followed by the urge to prescribe the instant and obvious cure'. Lay practitioners often find it difficult not to tell others what to do when placed in the client/practitioner relationship and this may be one of the reasons why some people take up the caring professions, namely 'a need to be needed'. The status afforded by the qualification may influence the performance and sense of power of the practitioner. This is equally true of health professionals, such as nurses and physiotherapists, who become reflexologists and who now appear to have an opportunity (which they may not have had previously) to consult, examine, make initial diagnoses and to select, perform and prescribe further treatments. (This does not apply to midwives, however, who are legally permitted to perform all of these elements within their own accountability for women with normal pregnancies.)

A 'prescription' is a 'written direction for the preparation and adminis-tration of a remedy' (Dorland's Medical Dictionary 1994). One would immediately think of the written instruction given to the patient by a GP who makes an initial diagnosis and selects appropriate treatment, giving the patient a written directive for medication. However, clinical reflex-ologists are qualified to 'prescribe' reflexology for their clients as a result of an assessment and to decide upon further treatments, although it is essen-tial that they acknowledge their professional boundaries. There is much debate regarding the issue of multiskilled professionals but short introduc-tory sessions on other therapies such as nutrition, which may be included in basic training courses, do not equip a reflexologist to work also as a nutritional therapist. On the other hand, if, because of such awareness of nutrition, a serious deficiency in a client's diet becomes evident during treatment, it would also be irresponsible to ignore this. If the practitioner is also qualified to provide nutritional advice, a separate appointment could be offered, as a change of 'hat' helps the client to identify the change of role. To monitor reflexology effectiveness without complication some reflexolo-gists choose to refer such clients to another nutritional therapist. Conversely, the combination of therapies can work synergistically for the client's wellbeing and should not be discounted, but the issues pertinent to this scenario are not discussed in this chapter.

'REFLEXOLOGISTS SHOULD NOT TREAT SPECIFIC CONDITIONS'

With regard to treating specific illnesses, the use of the terms 'treat' and 'cure' are often confused. When seeking clinical reflexology treatment prospective clients usually do have a specific condition in mind, but practitioners should neither guarantee a resolution of the client's problems nor go to the other extreme and, in an effort not to promise a cure, negatively imply that reflexology will not help them in any way. When clients present with a specific condition, such as back pain, complementary and conventional practitioners have the identical restriction in that neither can guarantee a cure. In addition there are certain legal restrictions on treating and curing: a practitioner cannot guarantee to 'cure' cancer, is prohibited from 'treating' specific conditions, such as sexually transmitted diseases and tuberculosis, and the care of pregnant and childbearing women should be carried out only by a midwife or doctor except in an emergency. That is not to say, however, that someone with any of these conditions should refrain from receiving reflexology, for many benefits to their overall sense of wellbeing can be gained from the physical, emotional and spiritual effects of the therapy on the whole person.

There is also a more contemporary issue at stake here, for those who pedantically hold on to the view that they do not treat specific illness will have a problem with participating in research where projects are designed with very specific parameters. Research titles such as 'the effect of reflexology upon people with multiple sclerosis' or 'a randomized controlled trial of premenstrual syndrome treated with reflexology' would not be possible if reflexology could not be related to the specific condition (White 1999). Reflexologists may, therefore, treat clients who happen to be suffering from specific conditions, but treatment will be within an holistic context where the client's own healing potential may be triggered by the treatment, thereby leading to alleviation in symptoms.

The rule regarding the treatment of specific illnesses relates also to those conditions that are considered contraindications to treatment. It is necessary for contraindications to reflexology to be universal in order to facilitate the integration of the profession into conventional health care. Dorland's Medical Dictionary (1994) defines 'contraindication' as 'any condition, especially any condition of disease, which renders some particular line of treatment undesirable or improper', in other words, treatment which may endanger the client, the practitioner, or anyone else potentially involved, that is, other clients. As with reflexology charts, lists of contraindications also differ between authorities but it is important to reiterate the need for individual reflexologists to acknowledge their personal limitations of practice. Some authorities grade contraindications into 'absolute' and 'relative' (Marquardt 2000). One 'Manual for reflexology' identifies the categories of 'potential to cause harm'; 'inappropriate' and 'could cause harm unless the therapy is done with appropriate cautions'. (Plummer 1997). There is a temptation to define lists of contraindications based on specific conditions, but none could be long enough to cover every eventuality. There is then a danger in assuming that any condition or situation omitted from a 'definitive' list of contraindications must therefore be safe. Therapists who are content to keep their reflexology at a non-clinical level will have a list of contraindications that is much longer than an 'expert' clinical reflexologist whose list is brief. This leads to an impractical paradox that therapists need to develop greater clinical diagnostic skills to apply this longer list in order to proceed with a non-clinical treatment.

The list resulting from Plummer's grading (1997) numbers 25 contraindications and yet still does not include three of Marquardt's (2000) 'absolutes' one of which is aneurysm, qualified by the expression 'if known'. This condition, like deep vein thrombosis, which is also often listed as a contraindication, may exist undetected for many years. The rationale for these 'absolute contraindications' is that the result of inappropriate reflexology treatment could be fatal, in the case of deep vein thrombosis causing the thrombus to move due to stimulation of venous return. It is difficult to balance the alleged potential fatal consequences with the qualification 'if known', which recognizes that there is a possibility of unknowingly working on a client with one of these conditions. Reflexologists routinely adapt treatments to each client and should consistently proceed whilst exercising caution, thus any condition or situation that can be safely handled by exercising these precautions or adapting a treatment is not a contraindication.

It appears that a factor influencing many of the decisions to label a situation as a contraindication stems from an unbalanced view of how reflexology works and an overzealous use of the word 'stimulate'. Reflex points or nerve endings at the point of contact are 'stimulated' by reflexology, in other words, it achieves a therapeutic response. However, this should more correctly be referred to as normalization, the promotion of homeostasis or homeodynamics (Solomon et al 1990). Greater understanding of this process should assist the practitioner in identifying pertinent contraindications.

For example, stimulation of the thyroid gland reflex may stimulate thyroxin release in the case of an under active gland but it has not been found to do the same with hyperthyroidism, that is, a normalizing process takes place (Ingham 1984). To overemphasize the idea of 'stimulation' can be misleading, resulting in unfortunate decisions in clinical practice based, perhaps, on a fear of exacerbating the client's condition. An example of this would be the decision not to treat people with cancer because of the fear of stimulating circulation and spreading the disease.

Case study 3.4   The diagnostic potential of reflexology – an extent, a limitation and the value of continuing professional development

A GP referred a newly delivered mother for reflexology for migraine and depression. Initial assessment identified a constant 'fuzzy' head condition, 'gritty' eyes and perpetual tiredness to add to her depression, and inspection of the feet revealed a Candidial infection of the toenail. During the next four treatments the reflex area for the thyroid gland became progressively tender and palpable. The reflexologist sent a letter to the GP advising blood tests for thyroid dysfunction. However, soon afterwards, further research during a programme of personal study caused the practitioner to appreciate that all the mother's symptoms, including the toenail infection, were signs of underactive parathyroid glands (indistinguishably in the same reflex area of the foot as the thyroid) and he contacted the GP again to suggest tests for parathyroid gland function, with subsequent positive results. Vitamin D treatment was commenced along with continued reflexology and the client quickly recovered and progressed. This demonstrates the integrated diagnostic power of reflexology and conventional medicine and the importance of continuing professional development.

This therefore identifies another requirement for practice: the need to use standardized language and standardized techniques within the therapy so that reflexology develops as a profession. One of the ways in which a profession is defined is the use of terminology specific to its practice, but until reflexologists employ the same language there remains the potential for communication breakdown and misunderstanding. Similarly, although individuals will develop variations in practice, techniques need to conform to professionally accepted norms, so that one practitioner's appreciation of 'stimulation' or other techniques is the same as another's. We look forward to the lead the Reflexology Forum will set in establishing a national curriculum from the now-completed National Occupational Standards (NOS) (Mills & Budd 2000). This will help establish standardization of the variety of language, techniques, 'rules', charts and lists of contraindications that at present cause confusion to practitioners, students, teachers and to clients.

CONCLUSION

In order for reflexology to develop further as a profession, to gain greater acceptance, credibility and reputation, it is essential to continue to challenge and debate traditional knowledge and belief. Relieving restrictions that originated from an era when there was little experience of clinical practice enhances the healing potential of reflexology. Integration into conventional health care will open doors and widen the opportunity for treating people with specialized conditions, so facilitating research and thereby further enhancing the profile of the profession. It is vital that practitioners keep up to date through continuing education. Equally important is that the authorities within reflexology practice and education continue to improve the collaborative communications now taking place (see Case study 3.4), without seeing them as a threat to their personal autonomy. Research into reflexology must take account of the variations in practice and theory so that the boundaries can be pushed back ever further for the benefit of clients, practitioners and the profession.

REFERENCES

Arnold M. Chi reflexology – guidelines for the middle way. Australia: Self-published; 2000.
Benner P. From novice to expert – excellence and power in clinical nursing practice. Menlo Park, CA: Addison-Wesley Publishing; 1984.
British Register of Complementary Practitioners. Code of practice and ethics. London: Institute for Complementary Medicine; 1994.
Collins Modern English Dictionary. Glasgow: Collins; 1987.
Dictionary of Medical Terms. Oxford: Helicon; 1994.
Dorland's Medical Dictionary. 28th edn. Philadelphia: Saunders; 1994.
Dougans I. The complete illustrated guide to reflexology. Dorset: Element Books; 1996.
Foundation for Integrated Medicine (FIM). Integrated healthcare – a way forward for the next five years? London: FIM; 1997.
Gillanders A. Reflexology – the theory and practice. Bishop's Stortford: Jenny Lee Publishing Services; 1994.
Gooseman-Legger A. Zone therapy using foot massage. Saffron Walden: Daniel; 1986.
Gore A. Reflexology. London: Optima; 1990.
House of Lords. Select Committee on Science and Technology, Sixth Report on Complementary and Alternative Medicine. London: HMSO; 2000.
Ingham E. The original works of Eunice D Ingham: stories the feet can tell thru reflexology and stories the feet have told thru reflexology. St Petersburg, FL: Ingham Publishing, Inc; 1984.
Kaye A, Matchan DC. Reflexology, techniques of foot massage for health and fitness. Wellingborough: Thorsons; 1978.
Kunz K, Kunz B. The complete guide to foot reflexology. London: Thorsons; 1984.
Lett A. Reflex zone therapy for health professionals. Edinburgh: Churchill Livingstone; 2000.
Marquardt H. Reflexotherapy of the feet. New York: Georg Thieme Verlag; 2000.
Mills S, Budd S. Professional organization of complementary and alternative medicine in the United Kingdom. Exeter: Centre for Complementary Health Studies, University of Exeter; 2000.
Norman L. The reflexology handbook. London: Piatkus; 1995 (First published 1989).
Plummer H. A manual for reflexology. Cardiff: 1997. Distributed by the International Therapy Examination Council (ITEC).
Solomon E, Schmidt R, Adragna P. Human anatomy and physiology. Florida: Saunders; 1990.
Stormer C. Reflexology – the definitive guide. London: Hodder & Stoughton; 1992.
Wagner F. Reflex zone massage – the handbook of therapy and self. Wellingborough: Thorsons; 1987.
White A. Reflexology research record. Unpublished paper prepared for the Reflexology Research Trust. Exeter: Department of Complementary Medicine, University of Exeter; 1999.
White A, Williamson J, Hart A, Ernst E. A blinded investigation into the accuracy of reflexology charts. Complementary Therapies in Medicine 2000; 8:166–172.
Wildwood C. The aromatherapy and massage book. London: Thorsons; 1994.

APPENDIX

MAP 1   FOOT CHART (©CLIVE O'HARA, 1981, 1991)

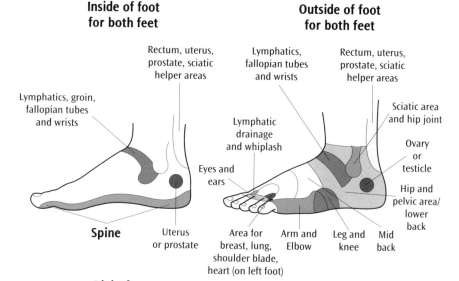

MAP 2   REFLEXOLOGY FOOT CHART (©CLIVE O'HARA, 1996)

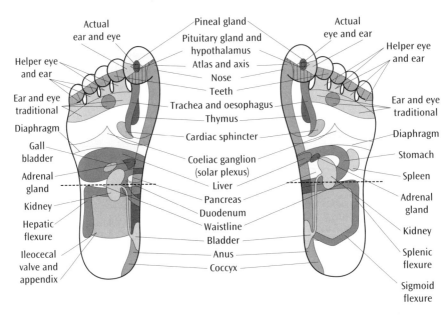

Right foot   **Left foot**

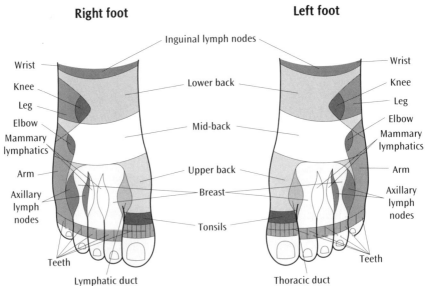

Map 2 is intended as a supplement and does not include all the reflex areas from Map 1.

MAP 3   REFLEXOLOGY HAND CHART (©CLIVE O'HARA, 1991)

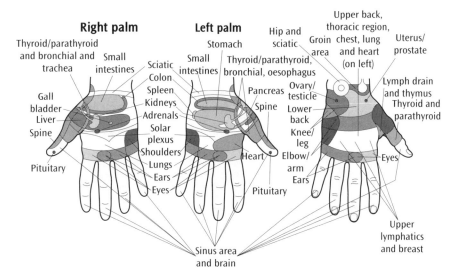

4

Identifying ethicolegal and professional principles

Julie Stone

Ethical and legal duties to benefit and not harm patients	Respecting the patient's autonomy
Beneficence and non-maleficence	Ethical requirements of the duty to respect autonomy
Competence and limits of competence	Legal facets of the duty to respect autonomy
Reflexologists' duty of care	**Conclusion**
Reflexologists who commit crimes	**References**
Maintaining safe, effective boundaries	**Further reading**

Abstract

Although few reflexologists are likely to be sued in the course of their professional practice, all practitioners owe their patients a duty of care and must work within the law. Ethical and legal responsibilities are integral to safe and effective practice. This chapter will outline the major ethical and legal responsibilities owed by reflexologists to their patients.

Key words: benefiting and not harming, confidentiality, consent, ethical and legal duty of care, limits of competence, respect for autonomy

The popularity of clinical reflexology has increased dramatically in recent years (Zollman & Vickers 1999). However, although there has been growing awareness of the therapeutic potential of reflexology, the ethical and legal issues facing its practitioners have received little specific attention, perhaps because of the assumption that reflexology is gentle, relaxing and considered to be harmless. Nevertheless, any therapy that has the capacity to benefit a patient also has the capacity to cause harm when used inappropriately. Ethical issues, such as seeking consent to treatment, respecting a patient's confidentiality, and maintaining appropriate boundaries, are as relevant to reflexologists as to any other practitioner, whether in complementary or conventional health care, and these ethical issues may also give rise to legal issues.

ETHICAL AND LEGAL DUTIES TO BENEFIT AND NOT HARM PATIENTS

BENEFICENCE AND NON-MALEFICENCE

Patients are entitled to expect that their therapeutic encounter with a reflexologist will be of benefit to them and, at the very least, will not cause them harm. These expectations (or rights) are encapsulated in the ethical duties of beneficence (benefiting) and non-maleficence (not harming), ethical principles that are at the heart of all healthcare relationships. These duties form the basis of most codes of ethics and are a central plank of Hippocratic tradition. As in most complementary therapies, the notion of what constitutes 'benefiting' in reflexology is somewhat wider than within conventional medicine. Whereas medical benefit usually involves the removal of symptoms, reflexology may benefit patients by preventing illness from arising or may improve the patient's mental outlook on his or her condition through the relaxation effect. The corollary is that harm may be caused during a reflexology treatment not just by physically injuring the patient, but by causing emotional damage or preventing the patient from seeking more appropriate treatment. Therapists must always avoid making inappropriate claims for reflexology, and indeed are bound by the laws pertaining to specific conditions, for example, not guaranteeing to cure cancer, not providing maternity care except in an emergency and not attempting to treat sexually transmitted disease.

COMPETENCE AND LIMITS OF COMPETENCE

To be able to benefit patients, reflexologists must be competent. Competence requires both technical proficiency and ethical literacy, that is, the ability to analyse and reflect upon ethical dilemmas arising in practice. As many reflexologists work single-handedly in private practice, therapists must recognize their own limits of competence and should, in the case of doubt, refer a patient onto someone better able to provide the necessary treatment – be that person a more senior reflexologist, another complementary practitioner, or a doctor. Accurate diagnosis is an important component of proficient practice and requires the therapist to recognize when the patient requires more intensive therapy than the reflexologist can offer. Reflexologists must also be in good physical and mental health in order to be able to treat patients effectively and safely.

The current common law allows freedom to practise, by which anybody can set up as a reflexologist (or other complementary therapist) without any training whatsoever. This makes it hard for patients to ascertain who is and who is not a competent reflexologist (Stone & Matthews 1996). Personal recommendation of 'good' practitioners may be a reasonably reliable means of finding a competent reflexologist, although this may simply be the subjective assessment of a previous patient who happened to develop a good rapport with the therapist. The general public should be encouraged, by the practitioner, to contact the reflexology professional organizations to confirm minimum training requirements and qualification of the individual therapist. The regulatory body will also be able to provide information regarding their Code of Ethics, which will determine the standard of professional behaviour expected of its therapists, as well as any complaints mechanisms that exist in the event of mishap. The coexistence of a number of professional registers within reflexology does little to ease the uncertainties facing patients or purchasers of reflexology, although this is changing.

'Best practice' demands not just high standards of pre-registration training, but also a commitment on the part of the reflexologist, once qualified, for continuing professional development (CPD) and, where possible, supervision of practice (Mackereth 2001). Reflexologists must be up to date with current research in order that practice can be based on contemporary evidence. With increasing governmental interest in complementary medicine (House of Lords 2000) the reflexology profession will have to invest energy and resources into research, because without evidence as to both the efficacy and safety of reflexology, it will be difficult to know for sure whether or not patients are receiving the best treatment possible (Ernst 1996).

REFLEXOLOGISTS' DUTY OF CARE

The ethical duty to benefit patients is mirrored by a legal and professional duty of care requiring practitioners to treat patients with all due care and skill. Reflexologists who fall short of their duty and cause patients harm may be found negligent if sued in a civil court, or may be liable to appear before a professional misconduct hearing. The most likely legal action against a reflexologist is negligence. Negligence may arise out of any sphere of a reflexologist's activities, such as failure to diagnose adequately or correctly, negligent treatment or negligent failure to disclose risks to the patient before providing treatment.

To be accused of negligence does not imply that the reflexologist intended to cause the patient harm. In determining whether a reflexologist had been negligent, the court would apply the Bolam test of professional negligence (*Bolam* v. *Friern Hospital Management Committee* 1957). This test of professional negligence states that the standard of care owed by the reflexologist to the patient is that which could be expected of a reasonably skilled and competent reflexologist acting in those circumstances. In ascertaining 'reasonableness', the court would look to national standards current at the time of the incident, such as National Vocational Qualifications, Occupational Standards or seek evidence from an expert witness. The absence of a single professional standard within reflexology at the time of writing presents difficulty in ascertaining the appropriate standard of reasonableness.

It is noticeable that the incidence of litigation against reflexologists arising out of their professional practice is minimal, and this is reflected in the low premiums for personal professional indemnity insurance which are paid by clinical reflexologists. It is possible, however, that as reflexology becomes more professionalized and better organized, the incidence of litigation may paradoxically rise. Increasing integration of the therapy into mainstream healthcare services will automatically result in a larger client caseload, thus reducing time and availability of the practitioner for each individual patient. Examples of possible reasons for litigation include situations in which practitioners fail to recognize that patients are more seriously ill than their competence permits them to treat; or failing to warn patients intending to return to a job in which they operate heavy machinery of the potential drowsiness following treatment.

REFLEXOLOGISTS WHO COMMIT CRIMES

It has already been stated that negligence involves unintentional harm. However, in criminal law, for a reflexologist to be successfully prosecuted for a crime, the crown prosecutor would have to show that the reflexologist both committed the criminal act and intended to do so. Examples of criminal offences include sexually assaulting a patient or stealing money from a patient. Falsifying one's tax return, for example by failing to disclose income from patients who paid in cash, would also constitute a criminal offence.

One would hope that few, if any, reflexologists would be prosecuted in connection with their professional practice. As well as having dire personal consequences for the practitioner, criminal acts within professional practice would breach the primary ethical principle to do patients no harm. They would also be a breach of the fiduciary relationship that is at the heart of the therapeutic encounter, in which the patient should be able to assume that the reflexologist will act at all times in the patient's best interests and that the patient will not be used as a means to an end, for example, that the reflexologist will not create a dependency on the part of the patient to satisfy his or her own need to be needed.

MAINTAINING SAFE, EFFECTIVE BOUNDARIES

Safe, effective therapy requires safe, effective boundaries. Practitioners should strive to create firm emotional, sexual and financial boundaries with their patients. Although reflexologists are no more likely to abuse the relationship of trust than any other health professional, evidence of professional abuse is, unfortunately, surfacing within almost all health professions. Moreover, the particular dynamics of the complementary and alternative medicine (CAM) relationship may increase the likelihood of boundary violation by both therapist and patients. A reflexologist's therapeutic concern and empathy may be mistaken by a vulnerable, or indeed manipulative, patient for personal or romantic emotional interest. If the reflexologist gives a welcoming or departing hug this could be misconstrued as a sexual advance. Similarly, overfamiliarity on the part of the reflexologist may cause the patient mistakenly to consider the therapist as a friend and to start asking personal questions that the therapist feels it is not appropriate to answer. The lending and borrowing of money to and from patients is almost always inappropriate and liable to lead to misunderstanding and bad feeling. Although it would be regrettable if, in order to prevent these problems, reflexologists felt bound to practise more defensively, practitioners must also be aware of the dangers of an allegation of abuse and take the relevant steps, such as the maintenance of detailed, contemporaneous notes, to avoid unfair or inaccurate accusations.

RESPECTING THE PATIENT'S AUTONOMY

Respecting autonomy means allowing patients to make decisions about their own lives and to act in accordance with their own set of values and preferences. Most reflexologists consider that they provide treatment that is individualized, holistic and ultimately patient centred. Certainly, one would hope that a therapeutic encounter in which the patient is given the time and space to explore his or her feelings at length, as well as discussion of physical symptoms, would facilitate the patient's involvement in the therapeutic process and increase their sense of empowerment. The reflexology patient is not a mere passive recipient of treatment. For reflexology to be maximally efficacious, patients have to be active participants in their own healing, making whatever adjustments to diet, exercise, stress levels or mental outlook the practitioner recommends.

Conversely, this does not mean that reflexologists are incapable of acting paternalistically, such as when practitioners believe that they 'know better' and seek to override the patient's wishes or fails even to elicit the patient's views. Such behaviour is rightly condemned within medicine as an abuse of the professional's power and is no more acceptable in clinical reflexology than in any other area of health care. In condemning paternalism, we must not, however, lose sight of the fact that some patients want their reflexologist to make some decisions for them. Some otherwise autonomous patients may luxuriate in allowing themselves to become temporarily dependent upon a therapist for a period of time. Nor is the patient's capacity for acting autonomously a prerequisite of the therapeutic relationship. Reflexology can provide benefit even when patients are not autonomous (e.g. where they are suffering from learning disabilities or are incompetent minors). What is important is that when patients wish to be autonomous reflexologists do not supplant patients' values and preferences with their own.

ETHICAL REQUIREMENTS OF THE DUTY TO RESPECT AUTONOMY

Most of the ethical requirements to do with autonomy concern information. To redress the power disequilibrium inherent in the professional relationship, the reflexologist must disclose as much information as the patient needs or desires to know in order to make an informed decision whether or not to proceed with treatment. This will include information about the therapy, how long each session is going to last, how many sessions are likely to be necessary, what the reflexology is likely to achieve and, if the patient wants to know, information about the reflexologist's training and therapeutic orientation. Patients also need to be informed of their obligations for the duration of the professional encounter. Respect for autonomy involves treating the patient as an equal in decision-making and keeping them informed and involved as the therapeutic relationship deepens. Consent, in particular, is not a one-off event, but an ongoing process.

Respecting the patient's autonomy also requires that the reflexologist treats as confidential any information given by the patient during the therapeutic consultation. Patients invariably disclose a significant amount of personal information in the course of their treatment. They do so trusting that this information will be used solely for their benefit. However, reflexologists need to be able to explain to patients that this duty is not absolute and that there may be rare situations when the reflexologist may be obliged to breach the patient's confidentiality (Case study 4.1).

Reflexologists should familiarize themselves with their professional code of ethics and be aware of the particular circumstances in which strict confidentiality may be overridden. This might include the legal duty on the part of the reflexologist to inform the local Medical Officer in the case of discovering that a patient has a notifiable disease or, rarely, if the patient tells the reflexologist something in the course of a treatment session that causes the reflexologist to fear that the life or safety of a third party is at risk. An example might be if the patient confides to the reflexologist that he or she intends to commit a serious assault on a named individual, and the reflexologist genuinely believes that breaching confidentiality and warning the individual will significantly reduce the likelihood of that individual suffering harm.

LEGAL FACETS OF THE DUTY TO RESPECT AUTONOMY

The law may protect a patient's autonomy in a number of ways. The civil action of battery (or trespass to the person) most closely protects the

---

Case study 4.1 An ethical dilemma

Jeanette had been receiving regular reflexology for a few weeks when she confided to her reflexologist that she was pregnant for the second time and that, because of her dissatisfaction with the first experience she had decided to care for herself during this pregnancy and that her partner was intending to deliver the baby at home without midwifery support. Jeanette did, however, wish to continue to receive reflexology throughout the pregnancy.

The reflexologist felt very concerned about this and discussed the case anonymously with her supervisor, who informed her that it is illegal for anyone other than a midwife or doctor to deliver a baby except in an emergency (see Chapter 10). However, the dilemma for the practitioner was being asked to continue the treatment in the knowledge that Jeanette was pregnant and at risk of complications as a result of her previous delivery. She could not be seen to be colluding with Jeanette's wishes and yet could not break Jeanette's confidentiality by referring her to the local midwifery service, which she had no desire to use.

The practitioner advised Jeanette that she would be willing to provide reflexology care during the pregnancy on condition that Jeanette sought the appropriate maternity support. Jeanette was given contact details of the local Supervisor of Midwives but declined to follow this up, so the reflexologist felt obliged to withdraw her services.

---

patient's bodily autonomy. A battery is occasioned when a reflexologist touches a patient, for example, in the course of physically examining the patient, without having obtained consent. Usually, a patient's consent to be touched may be implied if the patient lies down and makes no obvious objection to examination or treatment. Such consent would only extend to that which a reflexologist could be reasonably certain that the patient would agree to if asked directly. The concept of implied consent would not permit, for example, a vaginal or rectal examination as part of a physical examination, which, in any case, would be wholly inappropriate within standard reflexology practice, although it may be relevant if the therapy was incorporated into midwifery or gynaecological nursing practice.

Failure to provide information about the risks of reflexology might also result in an action for negligence. This might arise, if, for example, a reflexologist failed to warn a diabetic patient about the risks of treatment and the patient, consenting to treatment unaware of those risks, suffered harm as a result of the reflexology. However, this extends only so far as contemporary evidence available at the time.

Reflexologists are also under a legal, professional and ethical duty to respect confidentiality. Occasionally, a patient might be able to sue a reflexologist who disclosed confidential information learned in the course of the professional relationship, particularly if economic loss was sustained as a result of the unauthorized disclosure. Reflexologists must also comply with their legal responsibilities in relation to data protection, and ensure that their manual and computer records are maintained in accordance with statutory requirements. The Data Protection Act 1998 extends a practitioner's duty to safeguard certain manual as well as computer-based health records. Although reflexologists are not yet included in the list of professionals who are duty-bound to allow their patients access to their records by law, they should do this as a mark of respect for autonomy, and might even wish to consider providing patients with a copy of their records. Where reflexology is used within some other form of professional clinical practice whose practitioners are required to comply with these regulations, they apply also to the reflexology-specific data.

CONCLUSION

Reflexology is generally thought of as safe and non-invasive, and it may mistakenly be assumed that few ethical and legal issues arise. The purpose of this chapter has been to demonstrate that ethical and legal issues arise in all professional relationships and that the harm that an incompetent reflexologist may cause a patient need not be physical. The requirements of ethical and legal principles go beyond requiring that the reflexologist be technically competent. For clinical reflexology to continue to grow in credibility as an adjunct to mainstream health care, practitioners must be familiar with their ethical and legal responsibilities and accept that they are accountable to their patients, their profession and to society as a whole. As well as fulfilling individual responsibilities, reflexologists should take responsibility for the collective aspects of their profession, volunteering, for example, to participate in the profession's disciplinary mechanisms and mentoring colleagues who have recently qualified. Hopefully, adherence to the principles outlined above will ensure that reflexology continues to grow in reputation, respectability and credibility and that adverse incidents remain few and far between.

REFERENCES

Bolam v. *Friern Hospital Management Committee* 1957 1WLR 582.
Ernst E. The ethics of complementary medicine. Journal of Medical Ethics 1996; 22:197–198.
House of Lords. Select Committee on Science and Technology. Sixth Report on Complementary and Alternative Medicine. London: HMSO; 2000.
Mackereth P. Clinical supervision. In: Rankin-Box D, ed. The nurses' handbook of complementary therapies. 2nd edn. London: Baillière Tindall; 2001:33–42.
Stone J, Matthews J. Complementary medicine and the law. Oxford: Oxford University Press; 1996.
Zollman C, Vickers A. Users and practitioners of complementary medicine. British Medical Journal 1999; 319;836–838.

FURTHER READING

Cohen M. Complementary and alternative medicine: legal boundaries and regulatory perspectives. New York: Johns Hopkins University Press; 1998.
Dimond B. The legal aspect of complementary therapy practice. London: Churchill Livingstone; 1998.

5

Researching reflexology

Helen Poole

Existing reflexology research
  Case series/studies
Conclusion: future directions
References

Further reading
Appendix: Brief summary of
  research reviewed

Abstract

There is a plethora of anecdotal evidence to suggest that reflexology may be
effective for particular conditions, but little rigorous research evidence to support
this. This chapter explores the issue of research within the reflexology profession,
looks at the questions that should be asked and makes some suggestions for the
direction of future research. A review of some of the published reflexology research is
also included.

Key words: evidence, methodology, future directions

Interest in complementary and alternative medicine has increased rapidly
in recent years (BMA 1993, FIM 1997, House of Lords 2000) and reflexology has undergone a huge growth in popularity. There are an estimated
12 500 registered reflexologists in the UK, (Budd & Mills 2000) and the
prevalence of treatments ranges from 0.7% to 15% (Ernst & Koder 1997,
MacLennan et al 1996), with about 4.33 million visits per year (Thomas et
al 2001). There has also been an increased demand for complementary
medicine to be more widely available within the National Health Service,
and this has resulted in calls for evidence to support anecdotal claims of
efficacy (BMA 1993, FIM 1997, House of Lords 2000). However, the majority of reflexology research to date has been equivocal and not of a sufficiently rigorous nature to inform potential (NHS) purchasers of its clinical
effectiveness.

Many reflexologists claim to 'know' it works from the anecdotal evidence in everyday practice, and sometimes suggest that clients are not
interested in evidence (Coxon 1998), although others dispute this
(Cromwell et al 1999, Dryden et al 1999). However, for reflexology to develop further as a profession and become better integrated into conventional
health care, research activity is essential. Evidence of its clinical and cost
effectiveness, safety, modes of action and contraindications assist in

informing the general public, conventional healthcare professionals and NHS.

Not all reflexologists will have the desire or ability to undertake research and the 'scientist–practitioner' concept (Canter & Nanke 1993) may not be feasible for all practitioners, particularly those in private practice. However, for practice to be contemporaneous and of good calibre, practitioners should have access to the research findings of others and be able to interpret and apply them to their own professional work.

There has been relatively little research conducted into reflexology to date. Initially, research questions should focus on the safety and efficacy of the therapy, perhaps followed by investigations into its mode of action. Clients and professionals may want to know if the therapy is effective for a particular condition or, more precisely, if it is more effective, has fewer side-effects or is less expensive than a proven conventional treatment.

At the outset it is vital to develop a precise research question before determining methodology (Vickers 1996). The Foundation for Integrated Medicine (FIM 1997) has provided a framework to assist in the application of appropriate methodology to specific research questions that were adapted by Mackereth et al (2000) for reflexology (Table 5.1).

Table 5.1 Research questions and appropriate methodology to address them

Examples of research questions	Appropriate methods/design
Proving 'Is there a specific beneficial effect of reflexology?' (efficacy)	• Explanatory randomized controlled trial (RCT)
'How well does reflexology work in practice?' (effectiveness)	• Quasi-experimental design • Outcome studies
Improving 'Is reflexology a useful diagnostic test?' (developmental studies)	• Comparative study
Picturing 'Who uses reflexology and why?' 'Who provides reflexology and why?' (snapshots)	• Population survey • Purchaser and provider surveys • Focus groups and interviews
Understanding 'How does reflexology work?' (basic clinical research)	• Laboratory research • Explanatory RCT • Quasi-experimental design • Case studies
Developing research tools 'How do we assess the processes and effects of reflexology?' (outcome measures and instrumentation)	• Development and validation of measures and instruments • Cohort studies

EXISTING REFLEXOLOGY RESEARCH

There has been much criticism of the lack of rigour in methodology of reflexology research, with the inference that there is no evidence for the efficacy of the therapy (Botting 1997, Ernst & Koder 1997) although Graham (1999) suggests that the few research reports available appear to be positive, at least in the evidence for a relaxation effect, but also identifies the need for more carefully controlled studies. The acknowledged 'gold standard' methodology for clinical research is the randomized controlled trial (RCT), whereby the treatment under scrutiny is assessed against a control treatment, placebo or standard care to reduce bias. Random allocation of participants to alternative treatments ensures that the groups being compared differ only by chance, and thus any positive effects found can be more confidently attributed to the treatment received rather than the personal characteristics of the participant or therapist.

A data search for this chapter elicited nine published randomized controlled trials on reflexology plus numerous case studies/cohort series, and a few studies investigating its physiological effects, which while low in the hierarchy of evidence, do contribute to a conclusion regarding the efficacy of reflexology and identify areas for further study. A brief summary of the research reviewed in this chapter can be found in the Appendix, on page 72.

Siev-Ner et al (1997) conducted a randomized controlled trial to compare the effects of reflexology to non-specific calf massage on 71 multiple sclerosis patients, using paraesthesiae, urinary symptoms, muscle strength and muscle spasticity as the measurable outcomes. The reflexology group demonstrated significantly increased improvement in urinary and spasticity symptoms compared to those in the massage group, suggesting that reflexology was effective to some extent. Joyce & Richardson's study (1997) supports this, with a 45% improvement in symptoms of multiple sclerosis compared to 13% in the control group, although this benefit was not sustained at follow-up. However, whereas Siev-Ner et al's (1997) trial is considered to be methodologically sound, Joyce & Richardson's (1997) study has been subject to some criticism (Mackereth et al 2000) – participants were not randomized into the treatment or non-treatment groups and the outcome measures used were subjective.

Similarly, Thomas (1989) conducted a very small study that demonstrated the value of reflexology for anxiety compared with groups who had no intervention or simple reassurance. However, the lack of objective outcomes and the extremely small sample size identifies a need to repeat the study with a much larger sample using validated measures of anxiety before we can confidently surmise that reflexology is effective for anxiety. In addition, because human touch in itself can potentially reduce anxiety, this variable would need to be taken into account.

Oleson & Flocco (1993) used a particularly rigorous design to evaluate the efficacy of reflexology for 32 women suffering from premenstrual syndrome, by comparing reflexology with a placebo treatment that involved overly light or very rough foot massage on points not directly relevant to premenstrual syndrome. The women maintained diaries to record somatic and psychological symptoms on each day of the week prior to menstruation, which, before treatment, showed a similar number of symptoms in both groups. After treatment, a statistically significant ($p < 0.001$) 45% reduction in symptoms in the reflexology group compared favourably with the 20% decrease in the placebo group. As both groups were shown to have equivalent symptom levels before treatment began, the reduction experienced by those in the reflexology group can be more confidently attributed to the treatment. Furthermore, those in the placebo group thought they were receiving reflexology, which eliminates the placebo or non-specific effects. Oleson & Flocco (1993) speculate that the profound relaxation induced by the reflexology may have triggered a psychophysiological response to stress (Goodale et al 1990), which alleviated premenstrual symptoms, although Vickers (1996) points out manual pressure at the site of some classical Chinese acupuncture *tsubos* may have worked synergistically with the reflexology to influence the outcome. Ernst & Koder (1997) suggest that the therapist in this study may have been unconsciously biased, exposing the reflexology participants to non-specific positive effects such as expectation or empathy.

Two trials have investigated the use of reflexology for headache relief. Lafuente et al (1990) randomized 32 headache sufferers to receive either sham reflexology and Flunarizine™ (a drug used in the treatment of common migraine) or reflexology and a placebo. Participants recorded the frequency, severity and duration of headaches experienced. Over a 2–3-month period reflexology/placebo was shown to be more effective in reducing symptoms than sham reflexology/Flunarizine™, although the result is not statistically significant. Despite the relatively small sample size and variation in age and type of symptoms, it was concluded that reflexology was at least as effective as Flunarizine™ and may be a particularly appropriate alternative for patients with contraindications to pharmacological treatment.

Launso et al (1999) conducted a prospective, exploratory study of reflexology for headaches with a cohort of 220 patients who had previously received reflexology for headaches. Both qualitative and quantitative methods of assessment were used over a maximum 6-month period of treatment and a 3-month follow-up. Total relief was experienced by 23% and partial relief by 55% of participants. Those who had total relief also reported lifestyle changes and better understanding of their condition, which the researchers suggest resulted from the reflexologist acting as a catalyst for change. However, there was no control group or randomization in this study; no recognized outcome measures were used; and participants were self-funding, which may have meant a vested economic interest in the success of the reflexology treatment.

Vickers (1996), Ernst & Koder (1997) and White (2000, personal communication) have all reviewed Eichelberger's (1993) randomized controlled trial to determine whether reflexology could reduce the need for postoperative analgesia. All criticize the lack of experimental and statistical detail in the study report, in which 60 women catheterized while undergoing gynaecological surgery were randomized to two groups: reflexology versus no intervention. Eichelberger (1993) reports that only 10% of those in the reflexology group required analgesia after removal of the catheter compared to 40% in the non-intervention group. White (2000, personal communication) believes the subject is worthy of further investigation but Ernst & Koder (1997) argue that the design does not control for the non-specific effects of reflexology, therefore the results cannot be taken to demonstrate conclusively that reflexology was effective, as factors such as 'attention given' and 'expectations raised' in that group may have been responsible.

A study by Engwquist & Vibe-Hansen (1977) reported negative results on objective parameters. The study compared the effects of reflexology to the pituitary and adrenal zones with light reflexology to the shoulder zone for surgical stress, using changes in plasma cortisol levels as an outcome, and found no difference between the groups. However, the sample used was small ($n = 16$), and the reflexology was given for only 10 minutes prior to surgery. As most reflexology treatments last between 30 and 60 minutes per session, it may be that 10 minutes was insufficient to generate any effect, although Tiran (see Chapters 1 and 10) would dispute this.

Ernst & Koder (1997) review the English abstract of a study by Wang (1993) but note that the limited information available in the abstract prohibited a comprehensive evaluation. In this study, 32 patients with diabetes mellitus continued standard care but were randomized to receive either daily reflexology for 30 days or no additional care. Wang (1993) reports a return to normal levels of serum glucose in the reflexology group but not in the control group, suggesting a possible action of reflexology, although without comprehensive study details it is not possible to determine if other factors (such as changes in diet, or exercise) could have influenced glucose levels. In addition, time and financial commitments for daily reflexology may make this form of treatment prohibitive.

In Peterson et al's (1992) study, 30 patients with bronchial asthma were randomized to receive 10 weekly reflexology treatments or non-specific counselling. Outcome measures included diary and symptom scores, use of medication and objective intermittent measures of pulmonary function. No significant differences were found between groups, suggesting that reflexology is ineffective for bronchial asthma. Vickers (1996) notes that a single practitioner performed the treatment, thus it may have been the therapist, rather than the therapy, that was ineffective. Johannessen et al (1997) points out that the researchers' account does not correlate with that of the therapist (Fosholt 1992), whose evaluation of patient diaries concluded that reflexology was effective, although this is subject to bias.

This incongruence between results in the same trial presents an interesting dilemma when examining the evidence for efficacy. Peterson et al (1992) based their conclusions on objective outcome parameters but does not mean that patients' views of efficacy should be dismissed because they are in conflict with scientific findings. It is apparent, therefore, that outcome needs should be defined in terms that have currency and validity for both providers and consumers.

Poole et al's (2001) investigation into the efficacy of reflexology for 243 patients with chronic low back pain, using mixed methodologies, posed a similar dilemma. Qualitative results were evaluated by the researchers, rather than the therapists who provided the treatments. Patients were randomized to receive reflexology, relaxation or no intervention (continue standard care). Nine patients withdrew when the results of the randomization became known. The primary outcome measures were pain and functioning, measured by the SF-36 (Ware & Sherbourne 1992) and the Oswestry Disability Questionnaire (Fairbank et al 1980), respectively. Results revealed no significant differences in pain or functioning between groups, although all subjects experienced some reduction in pain. As with many longitudinal studies, subject dropout occurred, the greatest being in the usual care group, but additional analysis accounted for this and the results remained the same.

After the treatment phase 22 patients from the reflexology and relaxation groups were interviewed to ascertain the patient's view of efficacy. The majority experienced temporary pain relief, improved psychological wellbeing and an increased ability to cope with their pain, although these findings were not revealed by the quantitative measures. Patients may therefore be satisfied with qualitatively different, more subtle effects from treatment, which the 'objective' measures were not sensitive enough to detect. However, it is also possible that the interview data may have been subject to bias, for instance patients may have said what they felt the researcher wanted to hear. None the less, it is argued that patient views require consideration when selecting outcome criteria for research studies in complementary medicine.

The physiological effects of reflexology have been explored by Frankel (1997) who conducted a small, part-randomized study to determine the effect of a 45-minute session of reflexology on baroreceptor reflex sensitivity, blood pressure and sinus arrhythmia. Twenty volunteers were randomized to receive either reflexology or foot massage; another four volunteers acted as controls. There was no difference between the reflexology and foot massage groups, although both responded more than the controls. These results appear to indicate that reflexology is no different from foot massage, although it is not possible to determine if reflexology produced more than merely a relaxation effect because the control group may have introduced bias. Frankel himself accepts there are some limitations to the study, including non-randomization of the control group and the fact that he both delivered and evaluated the treatments. He suggests that repetition of the study with a larger sample and full randomization could address some of the limitations. However, as Mackereth and colleagues (2000) illustrate, an alternative approach would be to employ some form of quasi-experimental design.

CASE SERIES/STUDIES

Numerous case studies indicating the potential beneficial effects of reflexology for people with multiple sclerosis (Ashekenazi 1993), the terminally ill (Burke & Sikora 1992, Shaw 1987), expectant and newly delivered mothers (Tiran 1996), infants with colic (Wilson 1995) and those requiring pain relief (Lockett 1992) can be found, primarily in the literature of conventional healthcare practitioners who have incorporated reflexology into their practice, such as nurses, midwives and physiotherapists. These accounts and anecdotes may, of course, be subject to bias, as invariably they do not represent the whole case load. Vickers (1996) suggests that practitioners will submit for publication only their most interesting, most successful cases and that incidents of failure, less success or discontinuation of treatment will not be reported, although Mackereth (1999) and Tiran (1996) dispute this.

Trousdell (1996) evaluated the effect of reflexology to 15 women attending a drop-in mental health centre and suggests that its effects may be due to meeting the emotional needs of clients. Eight, weekly, 30-minute reflexology treatments were given to the women with open-ended semistructured interviews before treatment and at the end of the course, with the aim of eliciting participants' views of treatment effects. Three focus groups helped to validate the data. Trousdell states that many of the women reported physical improvements, including alleviation of back pain, premenstrual tension, normalization of blood pressure and increase in energy levels. However, the lack of a control group makes it difficult to accept that these self-reported improvements were solely due to the reflexology, and the analytic techniques utilized with qualitative data were not detailed. Nevertheless, patient perceptions are interesting, as they include both physical and psychological effects, highlight aspects which patients perceive to be beneficial and identify the need for more rigorous research in this area.

Coxon (1998) surveyed 18 patients who all reported post-treatment relief of symptoms, primarily back pain, with 10 also experiencing relief from other symptoms for which they had not sought help. Despite the small cohort and potential bias, some degree of patient satisfaction is apparent. This type of data is less robust than that from controlled studies but, used in conjunction, there appears to be some evidence for the effectiveness of reflexology, albeit non-specific. Anxiety reduction, deep relaxation and the therapeutic relationship may also be responsible for some of the positive outcomes experienced by patients, all of which are influenced by interindividual and interpersonal psychological factors, suggesting strong validity to the psychological theory of reflexology (as with other complementary therapies).

CONCLUSION: FUTURE DIRECTIONS

This chapter has reviewed some of the reflexology research conducted to date, highlighting several methodological problems and proposing some solutions. There is an urgent need to conduct more rigorous studies into both the efficacy and the safety of reflexology and, despite the 'gold standard' of the randomized controlled trial, it too has been subject to criticism (e.g. Poole et al 1999). Small preliminary studies are advocated in order to develop an evidence base as a rationale for larger studies and assist in successful applications of bids for funding.

However, it must be accepted that research activity is driven by more than a desire to answer pertinent questions. Several reasons for the paucity of research in complementary medicine have been mooted (House of Lords 2000), all of which apply to reflexology, including lack of funding, interest, training and expertise in research methodologies; lack of interest in complementary medicine amongst experienced researchers and inadequate tools with which to measure outcomes in complementary medicine. Individual practitioners/researchers may not be in a position to overcome some of these problems but reflexology schools and training institutions should henceforth include adequate training on research awareness, reviewing literature and examining research methodologies, enabling those wishing to remain in clinical practice to acquire the skills to evaluate research and incorporate findings into their practice, while those interested in conducting or participating in research would have a basic understanding of the processes involved.

The demand for evidence-based healthcare practice and the expansion of opportunities for the study of complementary medicine is an exciting dynamic which should be pursued (Mackereth et al 2000). Collaboration between therapists, between the NHS and the private sector and between complementary and alternative medicine is enabling a range of initiatives to be considered. Although reflexology research to date is of varying quality, the challenge now, for interested practitioners and researchers, is to respond to the criticisms and develop a programme of more rigorous studies.

A plethora of research questions needs to be addressed for reflexology to develop further as a discrete profession. It will not be an easy task, because clarifying some of the major issues, such as efficacy or mechanisms of action, will be a considerable undertaking. It will take time, in addition to research expertise and funding. However, it is only via the establishment of a firm research base that reflexology can hope to develop and expand its integration into mainstream health care.

REFERENCES

Ashekenazi R. Multidimensional reflexology. International Journal of Alternative and Complementary Medicine 1993; 11(6):8–12.
Botting D. Review of the literature on the effectiveness of reflexology. Complementary Therapies in Nursing and Midwifery 1997; 3(5):123–130.
British Medical Association (BMA). Complementary medicine: new approaches to good practice. Oxford: Oxford University Press; 1993.
Budd S, Mills S. Regulatory prospects for complementary and alternative medicine: information pack. Exeter: Centre for Complementary Health Studies University of Exeter on behalf of the Department of Health; 2000.
Burke C, Sikora K. Cancer: the dual approach. Nursing Times 1992; 88(38):62–66.
Canter D, Nanke L. Emerging priorities in complementary medical research. In: Lewith G, Aldridge D eds. Clinical research methodology for complementary therapies. London: Hodder & Stoughton; 1993:93–107.
Coxon T. Reflexology in the community. International Journal of Alternative and Complementary Medicine 1998; May:14–19.
Cromwell C, Dryden SL, Jones D, Mackereth PA. 'Just the ticket' – case studies, reflexions and clinical supervision (Part III). Complementary Therapies in Nursing and Midwifery 1999; 5(2):42–45.
Dryden SL, Holden S, Mackereth PA. 'Just the ticket' – the findings of a pilot complementary therapy service (Part II). Complementary Therapies in Nursing and Midwifery 1999; 5(1):15–18.
Eichelberger G. Study on foot reflex zone massage: alternative to tablets. Krankenpfledge-Soins Infirmiers 1993; 86(5):61–63.
Engwquist A, Vibe-Hansen H. Zone therapy and plasma cortisol during surgical stress. Ugeskrift for Laeger 1977; 139:460–462.
Ernst E, Koder K. Reflexology: An overview. European Journal of General Practice 1997; 3:52–57.
Fairbank J, Couper J, Davies J, O'Brien JP. The Oswestry low back pain disability questionnaire. Physiotherapy 1980; 66:271–273.
Fosholt U. Astma og zoneterapi. Zoneterapeutens beskrivelse af et astmaprojeckts for pa KAS Gentafte allergi -/ lungeklinik. Mit Helbred 1992; 10:18–21. Cited in Johannessen H, Launso L, Olsen SG, Staugard S. Studies in alternative therapy I, contributions from the Nordic countries. Denmark: INRAT & Odense University Press; 1997: 61.
Foundation for Integrated Medicine (FIM). Integrated healthcare: a way forward for the next five years? London: FIM; 1997.
Frankel B. The effect of reflexology on barreceptor reflex sensitivity, blood pressure and sinus arrhythmia. Complementary Therapies in Medicine 1997; 5:80–84.
Goodale IL, Domar AD, Benson H. Alleviation of pre-menstrual syndrome symptoms. Obstetrics and Gynaecology 1990; 75:649–655.
Graham H. Complementary therapies in context: the psychology of healing. London: Jessica Kingsley Publishers; 1999.
House of Lords. Select Committee on Science and Technology. Report on Complementary and Alternative Medicine, 6th report. London: HMSO; 2000.
Johannessen H, Launso L, Olsen SG, Staugard S. Studies in alternative therapy I, contributions from the Nordic countries. Denmark: INRAT & Odense University Press; 1997.
Joyce M, Richardson R. Reflexology can help MS. International Journal of Alternative and Complementary Medicine 1997; July:10–12.

Laufuente A, Noguera M, Puy C et al. Effekt der reflexzone behandlung am fuss bezuglich der prophylaktischen behandlung mit funarizin bei an cephalea-kopfschmerzen leidenden patienten. Erfahrungsheilkunde 1990; 39:713–715.

Launso L, Brendstrup E, Arnberg S. An exploratory study of reflexological treatment for headache. Alternative Therapies 1999; 5(3):57–65.

Lockett J. Reflexology: a nursing tool. The Australian Nurses Journal 1992; 22(1):14–15.

Mackereth P. Introduction to catharsis and the healing crisis in reflexology. Complementary Therapies in Nursing and Midwifery 1999; 5:67–74.

Mackereth PA, Dryden SL, Frankel B. Reflexology: recent research approaches. Complementary Therapies in Nursing and Midwifery 2000; 6:66–71.

MacLennan AH, Wilson DH, Taylor AW. Prevalence and cost of alternative medicine in Australia. Lancet 1996; 347(9001):569–573.

Oleson T, Flocco W. Randomised controlled study of pre-menstrual symptoms treated with ear, hand and foot reflexology. Obstetrics and Gynaecology 1993; 82(6):906–911.

Petersen LN, Faurschou P, Olsen OT, Svendsen UG. Foot zone therapy and bronchial asthma: a controlled clinical trial. Ugeskrift for Laeger 1992; 154(30):2065–2068.

Poole HM, Byatt K, Richardon C, Glenn S. The future of nursing research will be better served by mixed methodologies. Clinical Effectiveness in Nursing 1999; 3(3):103–105.

Poole HM, Murphy P, Glenn S. Evaluating the efficacy of reflexology for the management of chronic low back pain. The Journal of Pain 2001; 2(2):47.

Shaw J. Reflexology. Health Visitor 1987; 60(11):367.

Siev-Ner I, Gamus D, Lerner-Geva L et al. Reflexology treatment relieves symptoms of multiple sclerosis: a randomized controlled study. FACT 1997; 2:196.

Thomas M. Fancy footwork. Nursing Times 1989; 85(41):42–44.

Thomas K, Nicholl JP, Coleman P. Use and expenditure on complementary medicine in England: a population based survey. Complementary Therapies in Medicine 2001; 9:2–11.

Tiran D. The use of complementary therapies in midwifery practice: a focus on reflexology. Complementary Therapies in Nursing and Midwifery 1996; 2:32–37.

Trousdell P. Reflexology meets emotional needs. International Journal of Alternative and Complementary Therapy 1996; November: 9–12.

Vickers A. Massage and aromatherapy – a guide for health professionals. London: Chapman Hall; 1996.

Wang XM. Treating type II diabetes mellitus with foot reflexotherapy. Chung-Kuo Chungg Hsi I Chieh Ho Tsa Chih 1993; 13(9):536–538.

Ware JE, Sherbourne CD. The MOS 36 item short form health survey (SF-36): Conceptual framework and item selection. Medical Care 1992; 30:473–483.

Wilson A. A case of feet. Australian College of Midwives Incorporated 1995; 8(1):17–18.

FURTHER READING

Fitter MJ, Thomas K. Evaluating complementary therapies for use in the NHS. 'Horses for courses'. Part 1: the design challenge. Complementary Therapies in Medicine 1997; 5:90–93.

Lewith G, Aldridge D, eds. Clinical research methodology for complementary therapies. London: Hodder & Stoughton; 1993.

Thomas K, Fitter MJ. Evaluating complementary therapies for use in the NHS: 'Horses for courses'. Part 2: alternative research strategies. Complementary Therapies in Medicine 1997; 5:94–98.

Vickers A. Critical appraisal: how to read a clinical research paper. Complementary Therapies in Medicine 1995; 3:158–166.

Vickers A. A basic introduction to medical research. Part I: what is research and why do it? Complementary Therapies in Nursing and Midwifery 1995; 1(3):85–88.

USEFUL ADDRESSES

Centre for Complementary Health Studies
University of Exeter, Amory Building, Exeter, EX4 4RJ
Tel: 01392 264498
E-mail: CHS@ex.ac.uk

Reflexology Research Trust
4 Gordon House, 1 Gloucester Road, New Barnet, Hertfordshire, EN5 1RS
Tel: 07000 560432
E-mail: energyworks@clara.co.uk
Website: http://www.reflexologyresearchtrust.org.uk

Research Council Complementary Medicine
60 Great Ormond Street, London, WC1N 3HR
Tel: 0207 833 8897
E-mail: info@rccm.org.uk
Website: http://www.rccm.org.uk

Foundation for Integrated Medicine
12 Chillingworth Road, London, N7 8QJ.
Tel: 020 7688 1881
E-mail: enquiries@fimed.org
Website: http://www.fimed.org

APPENDIX   BRIEF SUMMARY OF RESEARCH REVIEWED

Study	Purpose/condition	Method	Treatment/ intervention	Primary outcome measures	Results	Comments
Eichelberger (1993)	To determine whether reflexology reduced the need for postoperative medication in a sample of women catheterized after gynaecological surgery	Randomized controlled trial ($n = 60$)	• Reflexology • No intervention	Need for medication	10% of reflexology group needed medication compared to 40% of those in no intervention group	No details of statistical analysis provided so not known whether differences between groups are statistically significant. However, suggestion that treatment with reflexology had some effect, although this may be due to attention given. More rigorous research required
Engwquist & Vibe-Hansen (1977)	To assess the effect of reflexology on surgical stress in patients undergoing cholecystectomy	Randomized controlled trial ($n = 16$)	• Reflexology to pituitary and adrenal zones for 10 minutes prior to surgery • Light reflexology to shoulder zone for 10 minutes prior to surgery	Levels of plasma cortisol	No differences between groups	No effect of reflexology. However, small sample and relatively short duration of reflexology treatment compared to that provided in everyday practice
Fosholt (1992) (therapist on the Peterson et al (1992) study)	See Peterson et al (1992)	See Peterson et al (1992)	See Peterson et al (1992)	See Peterson et al (1992)	Fosholt (1992) evaluated the treatment using the diaries and concluded that it was effective	Using different outcome criteria, reflexology appears to be effective. Methodological problems include bias on part of therapist evaluating own practice

Study	Aim	Design	Intervention	Outcome measures	Results	Comments
Frankel (1997)	To assess the physiological effects of reflexology on healthy volunteers	Part-randomized controlled trial. 20 randomized to reflexology or foot massage; 4 others included as controls (n = 24)	One 45-minute session of: • reflexology • foot massage • resting	Baroreceptors reflex sensitivity, blood pressure, sinus arrhythmia	No difference between reflexology and foot massage, but both responded more than controls	Suggests reflexology no different than foot massage. Not possible to say whether reflexology induced more relaxation than resting, as non-randomization of control group may have introduced bias
Joyce & Richardson (1997)	To evaluate the effects of reflexology for patients with multiple sclerosis	Non-randomized controlled trial (n = 27)	• Reflexology • No extra intervention	Patient ratings of 19 symptoms: minor/major/not applicable	45% of reflexology group reported that their symptoms improved compared to 13% of the control group	Suggests that reflexology had some effect on symptoms. However non-randomization could account for this as individuals may have had different levels of symptoms before treatment began. Also, results could be due to other factors such as attention given or the relationship with the therapist, as reflexology was compared to no treatment
Lafeuente et al (1990)	To evaluate the efficacy of reflexology for headache symptoms	Randomized controlled trial (n = 32)	• Reflexology and placebo • Sham reflexology and Flunarizine™	Diary of frequency, severity and duration of headaches experienced	No statistically significant differences between groups, although reflexology and placebo group improved more than the other group	Suggests that reflexology is at least as effective as Flunarizine™. Some methodological problems with the study. Needs repeating with larger sample to take account of variation in type of headache

Appendix (*contd.*)

Study	Purpose/condition	Method	Treatment/intervention	Primary outcome measures	Results	Comments
Launso et al (1999)	To determine the extent to which reflexology was effective for the treatment of headaches	Prospective, exploratory, cohort study with patients who had consulted a reflexologist (n = 220) In addition subsample, (n = 10) inter-viewed 3 months after treatment	• Patients were already attending reflexology treatment	3 months after treatment: • patient ratings (cured/experienced relief/no change) • analgesic use	23% reported cured, 55% experienced relief, 19% stopped analgesics	Indication that headaches may respond to reflexology treatment. Methodological problems: no control group or randomization, patients funded own treatment and no objective outcome measures. Further rigorous research needed
Olesen & Flocco (1993)	To evaluate efficacy of reflexology for women with premenstrual syndrome (PMS)	Randomized controlled trial (n = 32)	• Ear, hand and foot reflexology • Placebo (overly light or very rough massage on points not appropriate for PMS)	Diary of somatic and psychological symptoms of PMS experienced daily in the week prior to menstruation	At end of treatment reflexology group had 45% decrease in both somatic and psychological symptoms compared to 20% in placebo group	Indicates reflexology is effective for some symptoms of PMS. But foot reflexology was combined with hand and ear reflexology. Further studies required to assess foot reflexology, using larger sample size
Peterson et al (1992)	To consider the effectiveness of reflexology in the management of bronchial asthma	Randomized controlled trial (n = 30)	• Reflexology • No additional intervention	Medication use, pulmonary function, diary of symptoms experienced	No significant differences between groups at end of trial. Peak flow improved in all patients	Indicates reflexology ineffective for treatment of bronchial asthma. However, only one therapist delivering treatment, so perhaps therapist ineffective

Study	Aim	Design	Interventions	Outcome measures	Results	Conclusions
Poole et al (2001)	To evaluate the efficacy of reflexology in the management of chronic low back pain (CLBP)	Pragmatic randomized controlled trial (n = 234) In addition, subsample of those who received reflexology or relaxation (n = 22) interviewed after treatment	• Reflexology • Relaxation • Maintain usual care	• Pain (SF-36) • Functioning (Oswestry disability questionnaire)	Pain reduced for all patients. No significant differences between groups. Patients self-reported outcomes at interview, demonstrated that the majority experienced reduction in pain, increased relaxation and enhanced ability to cope with their pain	Quantitative results indicate reflexology is ineffective for the management of CLBP. Interview data suggests that reflexology and relaxation may be effective for some of the symptoms of CLBP. Incongruence between results raises questions for the design of research studies, particularly the choice of outcome measures, which requires further consideration
Siev-Ner et al. (1997)	To assess the efficacy of reflexology for patients with multiple sclerosis	Randomized controlled trial (n = 71)	• Reflexology • Non-specific massage of calf	Objective measurement of: • paraesthesiae • urinary symptoms • muscle strength • muscle spasticity	Significant improvement in urinary and spasticity symptoms for those in reflexology group	Indicates reflexology is effective for some symptoms of multiple sclerosis. Further rigorous research needed
Thomas (1989)	To determine the effectiveness of reflexology for reducing symptoms of anxiety	Non-randomized controlled trial (n = 9)	• Daily foot reflexology • No intervention	Patient reports of anxiety levels	Those in the reflexology group reported less anxiety than those in other groups	Very small sample size and lack of objective outcome measures. Indicates reflexology may be effective for reducing anxiety. More research needed using larger sample size, and recognized measures of anxiety

Appendix (contd.)

Study	Purpose/condition	Method	Treatment/ intervention	Primary outcome measures	Results	Comments
Trousdell (1996)	To assess the perceived benefits of reflexology reported by women attending a drop-in group at a mental health centre	Exploratory qualitative study (n = 15)	• All received eight, 30-minute sessions of reflexology	Participants were interviewed before and after treatment. Outcomes were self-reported benefits of treatment	Many women reported physical improvements and increase in energy levels	Interesting exploratory study. However, lack of a control group makes it difficult to accept that the reported effects were due to reflexology. They may have been the result of non-specific treatment effects, such as interaction with the therapist, or attending the drop-in centre. Further more rigorous research is needed in this area
Wang (1993)	To assess the effect of reflexology on patients with type II diabetes mellitus	Randomized controlled trial (n = 32)	• Daily reflexology sessions for 30 days • No extra intervention	Blood glucose levels	Blood glucose returned to normal in reflexology group but not in control group	Suggests reflexology may have had an effect on blood glucose levels. However, many other factors can influence this outcome, e.g. diet, exercise, medication. Further rigorous study required

6

Clarifying healing and holism

Peter A Mackereth

Abstract

Healing is frequently claimed to occur as a result of reflexology (Booth 1993, Griffiths 2001, Norman, 1989). There is a number of different perspectives of how this might happen, or indeed what 'healing' means. Dougans & Ellis (1995) suggest that reflexology helps to restore the body's balance of energy and thereby allows the body to heal itself. Arnold (2000) believes that reflexology can rebalance '*chi*' energy, empowering the receiver in his or her own healing. This chapter will explore definitions of healing and holism and how these terms relate to the clinical practice of reflexology. Essential to the discussion is the concept of spirituality, as an exploration of holism would be hampered without including this integral part of being human. Importantly for the patient and for the public who fund health services, outcomes need to be considered. Both healing crisis and healing responses are referred to in many reflexology texts; these too will be discussed. The practitioner, the therapeutic relationship and the space in which the interaction takes place will also be considered.

Key words: healing, holism, spirituality, connection, healing crisis, skilled companionship and healing environments

The term 'clinical reflexology' is used throughout this book to identify clearly its place and potential in health care. By prefixing reflexology with the term 'clinical' it might be judged that a case is being made for the practice to be viewed as a technical treatment. But pursuing greater integration in this way could be interpreted as a misguided attempt for respectability in the eyes of conventional practitioners. It could be argued that reflexology has a limited place in acute hospital care and that it is better suited to maintaining health and wellbeing (Lett, 2000). However, providing complementary therapies only outside acute healthcare settings ignores the reality of illness experience, whereby patients often move between primary care in the community and secondary and tertiary care in hospitals and hospices. Modern medical practice has been accused of being 'reductionist'

(Kendrick 1999) and, indeed, the popularity of complementary therapies (such as reflexology), can be seen as patients voting with their feet, looking for a radically different approach to healing. Nowhere is this more common than with patients experiencing chronic illness or enduring mental health problems. A study by Narayansamy (1996) found that a diagnosis of chronic illness was a pivotal life event and associated with an intense spiritual awakening, typified by the questions patients ask at these times: 'Why me?' 'Why now?'. An ill person may draw upon their family or friends for support, they may also seek spiritual guidance through meditation or prayer. Turning to help from complementary therapies is clearly a path for many patients faced with limited conventional medicine options. There is also a need by individuals to be treated as more than just another patient with a difficult illness or health problem.

HEALING AND HOLISM

People are more than physical and psychosocial beings and their lives and bodies are constantly undergoing change, some subtle, others dramatic. Although we share similar physical and psychosocial attributes and experience, for example, two feet, the need to eat and interact with others, clearly individuals have their own unique histories and hopes. Likewise, there are common patterns and responses to reflexology yet no two sessions are completely alike. In an attempt to create a systematic approach, assessment and treatment, guidance has been developed and indications and contraindications identified (see Chapter 3). The language of health and healing is inevitably constrained by how we see and want to be seen by other professions, the general public and how our own value judgement has developed through culture, experience and learning. Holism has become a popular, if not confusing term, to describe responding and working with an individual, mindful of their uniqueness. This approach is an attempt to promote individualized patient care in a healthcare system that, for pragmatic reasons, often manages and delivers care to diagnostic groups, such as oncology, intensive care, orthopaedics, rather than individuals who happen to have a particular 'Western' diagnosis. The complementary therapy movement has seized upon the term 'holistic', even attaching it to their titles and places of work. Arnold (2000) rejects the term 'holistic' because it might be linked with 'hole', meaning empty or lack of, opting instead for 'wholistic', coming from the word 'whole'. Gillanders (1994) claims that reflexology is a holistic form of healing, which aims to achieve a feeling of wellbeing by working with the mind, body and spirit. Norman (1989) claims that reflexology facilitates 'healing', that reflexologists are a channel for healing and that the work enables the body to cure itself. Kunz & Kunz

(1993) do not use the word healing, rather, they focus on the role of reflexology in relaxation and the regulation of physiological mechanisms leading to improved health. Dougans & Ellis (1995) suggest that reflexology can promote 'natural' healing by helping the body to rebalance and so enable self-healing to take place. Dossey (1995) has commented that the words, 'wholeness', 'healing' and 'self-healing' are often treated in the literature as though they were interchangeable terms. In the reflexology literature it is common for authors to make clear statements asserting that reflexology does not treat specific illnesses or symptoms (Dougans & Ellis 1995; Kunz & Kunz 1993, Norman 1989) and there is a general agreement that reflexology is but a means of supporting self-regulation and general wellbeing. In an era of evidence-based health care, identifiable outcomes for specific illnesses and symptoms are often essential prerequisites for attracting funding for an intervention. In exploring the potential of reflexology in healthcare settings, abstract notions of healing and holism pose a problem when exploring benefits and costs. One option is simply to back off and distance reflexology from conventional care settings; alternatively, a dialogue can be entered into concerning the meaning of healing. This could examine carefully both objective outcomes from research work, as well as asking patients about their own perspectives, of benefit, or otherwise of reflexology.

EVIDENCE FOR HEALING

Botting's (1997) review of the literature, presents evidence to support claims for healing that consist mostly of anecdotal reports from practitioners and patients. Small studies have reported positive effects on physical symptoms such as headaches, menstrual problems and constipation (Eriksen 1995, Lafuente et al 1990, Oleson & Flocco 1993). Botting (1997) suggests that these benefits may in part be due to expectation of improvement coupled by the 'quality and quantity of the personal contact between patient and therapist' (Botting 1997 p 125). Tiran (see Chapter 1) offers schools of thought regarding how reflexology works: these include an Eastern theory, whereby treatment areas relate to acupuncture meridians and Chi energy flow, and a Western theory, whereby helping to relax and de-stress recipients supports their innate ability to self-heal.

Trousdell's (1996) study reported noticeable 'reactions' to reflexology in 80% of participants. These included both emotional and physical responses. Examples ranged from one participant crying for 3 days, to many experiencing temporary increase in flatulence. The majority reported feeling relaxed and energized by the treatment, some participants perceiving a shift in attitudes and beliefs about themselves over the weeks of treatment. Frequently reported were feelings of being more able to cope, to focus better, improvements in self-esteem, greater confidence and a sense of being in control. One participant, as a result of the experience, described herself as 'blossoming into self discovery' (Trousdell 1996 p 10).

The effects of complementary therapies are cumulative, according to Penson (1998), who studied focus groups involving a total of 38 participants who accessed a service provided in palliative care. The therapies on offer included reflexology, massage and healing. Being able to express emotions and the quality of the therapeutic relationship were reported as even more important than the type of therapy. One client said when receiving her treatment 'I began to calm down a little . . . connect with my inner feelings and acknowledge my emotions' (Penson 1998 p 79). These studies begin to provide insight into the varied responses to complementary therapies such as reflexology.

REFLEXOLOGY AND THE HEALING CRISIS

The term 'healing crisis' appears regularly in reflexology literature; it is believed to be a short-lived response indicating detoxification (Griffiths 2001, Sahai 1993). Norman (1989) includes typical physical reactions of diarrhoea, nausea, headache and coldness. Griffiths (2001) lists similar responses and also reports that reflexology can affect the patient not only physically but also emotionally and spiritually. Norman (1989) also acknowledges that emotional reactions may occur attributed to 'energy' moving and relaxation. According to Norman, patients need only to be reassured that these symptoms will pass 'things have to get worse before they get better' (Norman 1989 p 94). These reactions could be quite disturbing for patients and may actually deter them or others who hear of their experience. Mackereth (1999), in exploring the concept of catharsis and reflexology, reports that patients have felt emotional, tearful and thought more about their lives past and present following sessions. For some individuals these responses, although initially alarming, may prove to be cathartic and beneficial. Recognizing catharsis and analysing whether in fact it is the same or different from a healing crisis, are important questions in attempting to critique the theoretical basis of reflexology.

Quinn (1989) explores the root of the word 'heal' and its origins in the Anglo-Saxon word *haelen*, meaning 'to become whole', suggesting that wholeness and relatedness are the same because they share opposites like 'alienation, estrangement and fragmentation' (Quinn 1989 p 140). It is suggested that awareness of fragmentation by the patient is an essential part of becoming whole. Essential to movement in this process is feeling, and being, safe in the therapeutic relationship. Reflexology affords opportunities through physical contact to be present with another as they engage with themselves and their lives. This is not only attributed to reflexology. Vickers (1996), reviewing the literature on aromatherapy and massage, concludes that these therapies, with their sensitive use of touch and an atmosphere of trust, can lead to 'emotional expression' (Vickers 1996 p 194). These kinds of experiences can lead to participating 'knowingly' in change (Cowling 1990). If becoming whole requires discharge of suppressed feelings then holistic interventions could be said to be working if catharsis occurs. It may be that the emotional component of a catharsis is not expressed and that only physical symptoms of a 'healing crisis' are reported.

On a practical level, it is important to recognize, manage and support a patient experiencing a healing crisis. Reflexology, in common with other complementary therapies, requires the practitioner to use interpersonal skills in supporting a therapeutic relationship (see Chapter 7). It is important to emphasize here that these interpersonal skills are not equivalent to those used in counselling or psychotherapy work. It also needs to be recognized that patients expect to receive reflexology and are not contracting for counselling or psychotherapy. There are many subtle and overt complexities to the therapeutic relationship. These include issues related to expectations, the space, the ritual and/or techniques employed and the quality of the contact between the client and practitioner (Elliot 1997, Freshwater & Biley 1998, Smucker 1998). Opportunities exist in touch therapies for self-awareness generated by receiving and engaging in a person-centred treatment that both acknowledges and works with the physical body (Westland 1993). These elements, when brought together, can have potent effects. It needs to be acknowledged that, for some individuals, being listened to by a perceived expert, whose focus is improved wellbeing through nurturing contact, can be a new and enriching experience. This would be particularly helpful if the individual's sense of self-worth is low or even absent (Gerachty 1992). For example, in Trousdell's study (1996) the participants – women who had been accessing mental health services – complained about being viewed as 'neurotics' by their doctors. Conversely, they reported being 'really listened to and heard by their reflexologist' (Trousdell 1996 p 11). The practitioner's demeanour, willingness to listen and use of 'quality time' have been argued as conducive to developing a therapeutic relationship, and to influencing patient responses (Wall & Wheeler 1996). Coupled with this is the need for a positive healing environment, which is both pleasant and relaxing (Biley 1996). An essential component to therapeutic work and relationships is a two-way dialogue with patients on their understanding of their illness, concerns, expectations and hopes.

Reflexology could also be said to be a therapeutic interaction that involves ritual. It usually involves a pattern of treatment and interventions to which patients become accustomed. Knowing what to expect can provide a space that encourages relaxation, and possibly time-out to reflect on feelings, plans, events and relationships. Freshwater & Biley (1998 p 73) state that ritual may 'actually expand the individual [practitioner's] connection to self, their clients and to their soul'. It also needs to be acknowledged that complementary therapies, with their lack of scientific basis, may in fact appeal to our imagination and be seen as a 'kind of magic' (Bell 1995 p 22). Hope and a search for meaning may lead patients to try reflexology.

SEARCH FOR MEANING: REFLEXOLOGY AND SPIRITUALITY

The National Association of Health Authorities and Trusts (1996) guidance on spiritual care suggests that everyone has a spiritual dimension and that this must be considered an essential part of holistic care. The health service has been labelled the 'illness service', given the ever-increasing demands limited by funding and staffing problems. The emphasis continues to be on maximizing efficiency in costs and time. Shorter in-patient stays and often hurried contact with members of staff can undermine relationships and the sense of being cared for. To form a relationship requires willingness and receptivity for both partners. Doing things for patients is not necessarily the same as 'being with' them. Spiritual care requires the practitioner and the patient to make and sustain a meaningful connection, which is often difficult given the time pressures of conventional health care. In a hospital-based reflexology study, Cromwell et al (1999) reported patient's appreciation of sessions, which, due to workload pressures, were limited to 30 minutes. Patients are perhaps drawn to reflexology in private practice precisely because they can be assured of time and privacy. If the subsequent relationship is to be holistic then issues related to spirituality need to be acknowledged by the reflexologists, wherever they are working.

Spirituality has been identified with a personal search for purpose and meaning (Walter 1997). A participant in a study by White (2000) described spirituality in terms of 'connection' to something else. This connection was further clarified as an 'integrated or holistic understanding of human nature, as well as relationships with other human beings, with the environment and – for some – with a divine power' (White 2000 p 482). In examining the origins of the word 'spirit' Goldberg (1998) acknowledges that the Hebrew word for spirit *Ruah* translates as wind, exhalation and breath. The abstract noun 'spirituality' has come to be associated with the non-material, otherworldly and non-physical. If the Hebrew definition is used, then it can be thought of as connected with the body and the essential processes of life. This can clearly be seen in the practice of reflexology, wherein the practitioner engages with the person by holding their feet and incorporating breath work; the common practice of solar plexus breathing. Goldberg (1998) explored the concept of spirituality and professional care and concluded that the essential component was 'connection'.

Working with the concept of spirituality within a reflexology session might be perceived as difficult to do or maybe even inappropriate. Stoll's (1979) four

---

Box 6.1 Stoll's (1979) guidelines: four areas of concern and sample questions

1. Concept of God or deity – how would you describe your God or what you worship?
2. Sources of strength and hope – what is your source of strength and hope?
3. Spiritual practices – do you feel your faith and religion is helpful to you now?
4. Relationship between spiritual beliefs and health – is there anything that is especially frightening or meaningful to you now?

---

areas of concern and sample questions are a useful starting point in clarifying our understanding of the patient's current situation and requirements (Box 6.1). Mackereth (2000) also proposes a model of contracting for complementary therapies that includes an energetic component (see Chapter 9) that can be related to a patient's preferred concept of energy or spirit.

THE PRACTITIONER: WORKING WITH HEALING AND SPIRITUAL ISSUES

In healing and holism it is important to explore what motivates healthcare workers, such as nurses and midwives, who work in demanding practice settings, to want to help others by offering reflexology. The purpose of nursing, for example, has been described as promoting 'health and wellbeing' (Rogers 1988). Yet as Coxon (1990 p 35) states, the 'very nature of nursing evokes stress and anxiety'. Dealing with people who are either experiencing acute illness or enduring chronic healthcare problems against a background of finite resources, including staff shortages, can be demoralizing and stressful. Added dissatisfaction with the alienation of technology and a market-driven approach to healthcare has led increasing numbers of nurses and midwives to complementary therapies in their search to 'enrich and deepen their contact with patients' (Elliott 1997 p 81). However, reflexologists need to be careful in assuming that all complementary therapists live and practise by a creed of holism. It is also important not to assume that all practitioners of conventional medicine are unwilling to consider alternative and complementary therapies. Some patients may be more comfortable with a pragmatic conventional healthcare practitioner than with a reflexologist who may use terms like '*chi-energy*' or incorporates work with the chakras. Of course, patients may have similar beliefs and could be drawn to a practitioner because of their views towards healing and spirituality. Campbell (1984) has talked about practitioners journeying with patients as skilled companions, a relationship that is committed but has clear boundaries, for the protection of both the practitioner and patient. This includes respecting, and even having reverence towards, the beliefs of others, for example, working with the patient's view of energy and healing (Case study 6.1).

For practitioners to sustain effective therapeutic relationships, reflective practice, clinical supervision and being open to the journey of personal

---

Case study 6.1 Working with the patient

Mary attended a hospital clinic that offered complementary therapies. She presented with altered sensation and pain in her arms and back associated with multiple sclerosis. Massage was her preferred option as she was sceptical about reflexology and also thought her priest would think it wasn't the right thing to do. Unfortunately, Mary found even the lightest massage work too painful. In talking to Mary I explained that there were different theories about how reflexology might work and that I would be respectful of her religious views. She agreed to give it a go. Mary continues to come for reflexology and reports that it helps with symptoms and general wellbeing.

---

growth and development are recommended (Mackereth 1997). Developing an affirmation statement such as the one below may be useful for staying focused and present in therapeutic relationships:

> [to have] . . . an open heart, a willingness to journey with others, but acknowledge that I have my own needs and issues for which I require support. I believe healing can take place if I can be with others and be myself in a way that defines our boundaries and helps to create sacred space for shared healing'
> (Mackereth 1998 p 127)

It would appear that patients, faced with illness and disability, experience an emergence of hidden or even repressed emotion when their bodies receive nurturing and support in a safe and therapeutic space. Crucially from a healing perspective, these responses can be powerfully cathartic, especially when witnessed and acknowledged by another, whose compassion and willingness to be present is clearly evident. It has been suggested that a practitioner needs to bring the 'three P's' to their therapeutic work. These are potency, protection and permission (Crossman 1966) and have been used as a framework to explore practice issues in clinical supervision (Mackereth 1997). First, patients need to know and feel that their practitioners are 'potent' in their work, to feel confident and trusting of their skills. Potency for practitioners is having and acknowledging specialized skills developed and sustained by being open to learning (Stewart 1989). Second, being clear about what the contract for the work is can help to develop 'protection' for both patient and practitioner (Stewart 1989). In reflexology this would include arrangements for making and cancelling appointments. For the practitioner this includes maintaining patient confidentiality within discussed limits (see Chapter 4). Importantly, in raising the potential for a healing crisis, the reflexologist would want to be informed of any physical or emotional responses to the treatment. Finally, patients need 'permission' – to know that it is 'okay' to give feedback about the treatment, to relax and enjoy the space offered by reflexology and to express how they are feeling. There are many and varied ways of maintaining the reflexologist's soul (Box 6.2).

Box 6.2 Maintenance of the reflexologist's soul

- Engaging in supportive supervision
- Joining/establishing a reflexologists' peer support group
- Participating in reflexology workshops and conferences
- Treating your work/life challenges as puzzles rather than problems
- Receiving reflexology and/or other complementary therapies regularly
- Praying or meditating on a daily basis
- Creating a working space that is a joy to work in
- Absorbing and giving praise for appreciated service/work
- Spending time enjoying and being with nature
- Eating healthy food and drinking plenty of water
- Finding an exercise/creative activity that brings you pleasure at least twice a week

---

SACRED SPACE: ENVIRONMENTS FOR HEALING

It is important to acknowledge that the increased integration of complementary therapies, and in particular reflexology, is part of a larger movement of increased public interest in health and wellbeing. It is also important to recognize that in a largely secular society many people are unsure about religious practices or what spirituality means to them. Conventional medicine has its limitations and, in times of crisis or when facing a future living with chronic illness, the material may offer little, if any, meaningful comfort. In the past, religion perhaps played a much larger role. As we enter the third millennium, with its technological advances but huge environmental concerns, values and beliefs are once more being discussed: the profits of industry are competing with the needs and habitats of indigenous people, the welfare of animals and the limits of medicine as cloning and gene therapy become a reality. This chapter has so far focused on the patient and the practitioner but healing, holism and spirituality are global, if not universal concepts. Engaging in reflexology could be seen as a peripheral matter but it does provide a space to receive nurturing and support, as well as physical contact.

On a macroscopic level, the movement to embrace complementary therapies with their emphasis on holistic care, not only challenges technological approaches to illness management but also provides choices. Medicine has been criticized for its paternalism, which, while well meaning, can be experienced as disempowering, preventing an individual taking responsibility and ownership of their bodies, lives, families and communities (Illich 1979). Nowhere is this more evident than in the care of women in childbirth (Oakley 1984). The work of Tiran (1996) and other innovative midwives working to integrate complementary therapies, offers choices and alternative strategies in managing what is largely a normal healthy process (see Chapter 10). The hospice movement has also been instrumental in providing an increasing range of complementary therapies to patients and their families at the other end of the life continuum (see Chapter 14). This movement also leads the way in creating environments that challenge our image of clinical and aesthetic utilitarian spaces. Hospital arts projects, the inclusion of pets, music therapy, the use of ambient lighting, colour and furnishings, can all contribute to nurturing the spirit and enhancing the process of healing (Fig. 6.1). Stone (2000) reminds us that the Greeks had a network of healing temples, often located in 'beautiful natural surroundings' (Stone 2000 p 39). Stone suggests that in enhancing clinics and hospitals, elements of nature can be included in waiting areas, therapy spaces, offices and patients' bedsides. This can include small water fountains, as well as plants and pictures depicting the beauty of nature. Designing buildings and placing objects utilizing Feng Shui, an ancient Chinese energy discipline, has attracted much interest in the West. Pauline Jeffreys, a Feng Shui consultant, suggests many ways to improve the energy balance of healing spaces, these include the use of fresh flowers; removing dried flowers and unhealthy plants; and careful selection and placement of furniture, wind chimes, water features and sources of light (Jeffreys 2000).

A therapeutic environment touches not only the lives of the patients and their families, but also those of the staff. Healing is a shared experience that, to be truly holistic, must extend beyond the confines of hospitals and clinics and reach into every part of the community. Reflexology is a part of that process, and its integration into a variety of healthcare areas is an important contribution to supporting health and wellbeing. Wright (2000) suggests that there are no healers or healees, and that we are all just in the work of healing together.

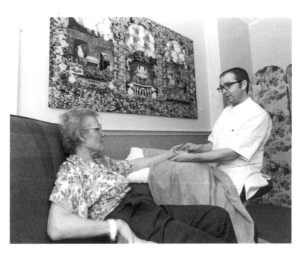

Figure 6.1 Patient receiving hand reflexology in a relaxation room reproduced with permission from Mackereth P. Journal of Complementary Therapies in Nursing and Midwifery 1999; 5(3):68

CONCLUSIONS

There are different theories about how reflexology might contribute to healing and healing responses. Catharsis has been proposed here as a niche in a theory of reflexology, whereby the therapeutic relationship and the nurturing physical contact play a valuable and significant part in outcomes for patients. It is claimed here that these elements can facilitate emotional discharge, coping and self-discovery, and that they can potentially revise beliefs about self-esteem. Reflexologists may 'know' and 'do' reflexology but they also need to 'be' with patients. It is acknowledged here that a period of regular and intense contact, with the focus on the individual, may also be a form of ritualized relaxation. Mind, body and spirit require healing together, affirming the commercial mantra 'because I'm worth it'. How much of the potential benefits to healing can be attributed to the therapeutic relationship, the environment or the application of pressure to a specific reflexology point or zone remains to be explored through further research work. It is very likely that compassionate practitioners, who are supported in their work, can help patients in their own healing. Integral to a holistic or wholistic approach is an appreciation that the spirit requires nurturing for the patient and the practitioner too.

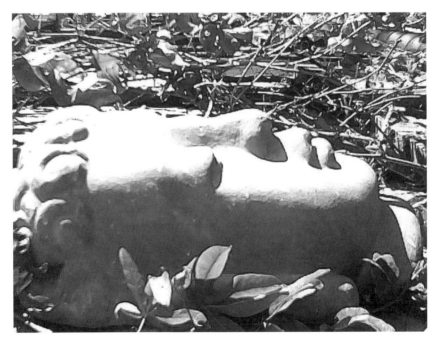

Photograph taken by Peter Mackereth

REFERENCES

Arnold MM. Chi-reflexology: guidelines for the middle way. Australia: Moss M Arnold Publications; 2000.
Bell W. Relax on reflexology. Nursing Times 1995; 91(2):22.
Biley F. Hospitals: healing environments? Complementary Therapies in Nursing and Midwifery 1996; 2(2):110–115.
Booth B. Complementary therapies. London: Nursing Times/Macmillan Press; 1993.
Botting D. Review of the literature on the effectiveness of reflexology. Complementary Therapies in Nursing and Midwifery 1997; 3(5):123–130.
Campbell A. Moderated love: a theology of professional care. London: SPCK; 1984.
Cowling WR III. A template for unitary pattern-based nursing practice. In: Barrett EAM, ed. Visions of Roger's science-based nursing. New York: National League for Nursing; 1990.
Coxon T. Ritualised repression. Nursing Times 1990; 86(31):35–37.
Cromwell C, Dryden S, Jones D, Mackereth P. 'Just the ticket': case studies, reflections and clinical supervision (Part III). Complementary Therapies in Nursing and Midwifery 1999; 5(2):42–45.
Crossman P. Permission and protection. Transactional Analysis Bulletin 1966; 5(19):152–154.
Dossey BD. Visions of healing. In: Dossey BD, Keegan L, Guzzetta CE, Kolkmeier LE, eds. Holistic nursing: a handbook for practice. 2nd edn. Gaitherburg, MD: Aspen Publications; 1995.
Dougans I, Ellis S. The art of reflexology: a step-by-step guide. Shaftesbury, Dorset: Element Books; 1995.
Elliot H. Holistic nursing and the therapeutic use of self. Complementary Therapies in Nursing and Midwifery 1997; 3(3):81–82.
Eriksen L. Using reflexology to relieve chronic constipation: A collection of articles. Denmark: Danish Reflexologists Association; 1995.
Freshwater D, Biley F. Rituals: the soul purpose. Complementary Therapies in Nursing and Midwifery 1998; 4(3):73–76.
Gerachty A. Counselling skills for practitioners. International Journal of Alternative & Complementary Medicine 1992; October: 10–11.
Gillanders A. Reflexology – the theory and practice. Bishop's Stortford: Jenny Lee Publishing Services; 1994.
Goldberg B. Connection: an exploration of spirituality in nursing care. Journal of Advanced Nursing 1998; 27:836–842.
Griffiths P. Reflexology. In: Rankin-Box D, ed. The nurse's handbook of complementary therapies. 2nd edn. London: Harcourt Publishers; 2001.
Illich I. Limits to medicine. London: Marion Boyars; 1979.
Jeffreys P. Feng Shui for the health sector: harmonious buildings, healthier people. Complementary Therapies in Nursing and Midwifery 2000; 6(2):61–65.
Kendrick K. Challenging power, autonomy and politics in complementary therapies; a contentious view. Complementary Therapies in Nursing and Midwifery 1999; 5:77–81.
Kunz K, Kunz B. The complete guide to foot reflexology (revised edn.) Albuquerque, New Mexico: Reflexology Research; 1993.
Lafuente A, Nouera M, Puy C et al. Effects of treatment with stimulation of the reflex zones of the foot with regard to the prophylactic Flunarizin™ treatment of patients suffering from headaches. In: Reflexology Research Reports. 4th edn. London: Association of Reflexologists; 1997: 39–40.
Lett A. Reflex zone therapy for health professionals. London: Churchill Livingstone; 2000.
Mackereth P. Clinical supervision for 'potent' practice. Complementary Therapies in Nursing and Midwifery 1997; 3(2):38–42.
Mackereth P. Body, relationship and sacred space. Complementary Therapies in Nursing and Midwifery 1998; 4(5):125–127.

Mackereth P. An introduction to catharsis and the healing crisis in reflexology. Complementary Therapies in Nursing and Midwifery 1999; 5(3):67–74.

Mackereth P. Tough places to be tender: contracting for happy or 'good enough' endings in therapeutic massage/bodywork. Complementary Therapies in Nursing and Midwifery 2000; 6(3):111–115.

Narayanasamy A. Spiritual care of chronically ill patients. British Journal of Nursing 1996; 5(7):411–416.

National Association of Health Authorities and Trusts. Spiritual Care in the NHS. Birmingham: NAHAT; 1996.

Norman L. The reflexology handbook. London: Piatkus; 1989.

Oakley A. Women confined. Oxford: Martin Robertson; 1984.

Olesen T, Flocco W. Randomised controlled study of pre-menstrual symptoms treated with ear, hand and foot reflexology. Obstetrics and Gynaecology 1993; 82(6):906–911.

Penson J. Complementary therapies: making a difference in palliative care. Complementary Therapies in Nursing and Midwifery 1998; 4(3):77–81.

Quinn J. Healing: the emergence of right relationship. In: Carlson R, Shield B, eds. Healers on healing. New York: The Putnam Publishing Group; 1989.

Rogers M. Nursing science and art: a perspective. Nursing Science Quarterly 1988; 1:99–102.

Sahai I. Reflexology — its place in modern health care. Professional Nurse 1993; 18:722–725.

Smucker C. Nursing, healing and spirituality. Complementary Therapies in Nursing and Midwifery 1998; 4(4):95–97.

Stewart I. Transactional analysis counselling in action. London: Sage Publications; 1989.

Stoll R. Guidelines for spiritual assessment. American Journal of Nursing 1979; 79:1574–1577.

Stone V. Designing environments to nurture the spirit. Sacred Space: The International Journal of Spirituality and Health 2000; 1(4):38–44.

Tiran D. The use of complementary therapies in midwifery practice: a focus on reflexology. Complementary Therapies in Nursing and Midwifery 1996; 2(2):32–37.

Trousdell P. Reflexology meets emotional needs. International Journal of Alternative and Complementary Medicine 1996; November: 9–12.

Vickers A. Massage and aromatherapy – a guide for health professionals. London: Chapman & Hall; 1996.

Wall M, Wheeler S. Benefits of the placebo effect in the therapeutic relationship. Complementary Therapies in Nursing and Midwifery 1996; 2(6):160–163.

Walter T. The ideology and organization of spiritual care: three approaches. Palliative Medicine. 1997; 11:21–30.

White G. An inquiry into the concepts of spirituality and spiritual care. International Journal of Palliative Nursing 2000; 6(10):479–484.

Wright S. Making a spectacle of a miracle. Sacred Space: The International Journal of Spirituality and Health 2000; 1(4):1–6.

FURTHER READING

Dossey L. Healing words. San Francisco: Harper; 1993.

Graham H. Complementary therapies in context – the psychology of healing. London: Jessica Kingsley; 1999.

Talbot M. The holographic universe. New York: Harper Collins; 1991.

Tingle J. Patient consent; the issues. Nursing Standard 1990; 21, 5(9):52–54.

Westland G. Massage as a therapeutic tool, Part 1. British Journal of Occupational Therapy 1993; 56(4):129–134.

Wright SG, Sayre-Adams J. Sacred space – right relationship and spirituality in healthcare. Edinburgh: Harcourt Brace; 2000.

USEFUL ADDRESSES

Art for Health
Manchester Metropolitan University, All Saints, Oxford Road, Manchester, M15 6BY

Sacred Space Foundation
Highland Hall, Renwick, Penrith, Cumbria, CA10 1JL
Tel: 01768 898375 377

Feng Shui Society UK
377 Edgware Road, London, W2 1BT
Tel: 07050 289 200
E-mail: info@fengshuisociety.org.uk

ACKNOWLEDGEMENTS

With thanks to Margaret Thorlby, who helped in the initial development of this chapter.

7

Exploring the therapeutic relationship

Margaret Thorlby and Cliff Panton

Principles of the therapeutic **relationship** **Client–therapist interaction** **Models for therapeutic relationships**	A model for reflexology practice **Conclusion** **References**

Abstract

Establishing a relationship between the practitioner and a client should be considered paramount and central to the therapeutic encounter (Mitchell & Cormack 1998). When such an encounter generates trust and confidence, it forms the basis for a positive therapeutic process and outcome. The therapist and the client must both be prepared to participate in the relationship, although there may by anticipatory anxiety and concerns on both sides. This chapter explores the value of the therapeutic relationship as an essential part of reflexology treatment. It will consider the quality of the relationship within the therapeutic milieu and the concepts of partnership and empowerment as essential components of a model for clinical reflexology.

Key words: therapeutic relationship, model for practice, partnership, empowerment

The aim of any therapeutic interaction should be to benefit the client through empowerment. Marchione (1993 p 13) refers to a 'person–environment interaction', which is enhanced by sensitivity and natural warmth of the therapist, thus contributing towards the client's sense of health and wellbeing. Liossi & Mystakidou (1997) suggest that provision of conditions that enable clients to determine their true needs, including the essential need to sustain a healthy lifestyle, will result in greater cooperation and thus a more successful outcome to the therapeutic interaction. Khan (1997) suggests that combining the whole ethos of care with the therapist's expertise and experience can help to create understanding and empathy for individual clients. Continuing professional development and reflective practice enable the reflexologist to achieve a sound level of expertise leading to improved self-awareness and competence as a practitioner, thereby recognizing capabilities, prejudices and limitations as factors that strongly influence relationships (Hill 1998). The therapeutic process is a partnership that enables individuals to regain control over their health and wellbeing and to progress towards independence.

A common and often dismissive criticism of complementary and alternative medicine by established orthodoxy is that there is no scientific proof to support its efficacy. Accordingly, any reported positive results are attributed to the placebo effect or simply to the time spent with the client. Healthcare professionals often remark that they do not have enough time to spend with patients. Chard et al (1999) argue that the 'creeping medicalisation' of normal experiences such as childbirth and death, and, increasingly, surveillance of health behaviour resulting in the separation of the mechanical and spiritual basis of healing, have been a source of much criticism. These views acknowledge the importance of time for nurturing within every care setting, which is equally important to the therapeutic relationship between reflexologists and their clients. With increasing access to healthcare information, consumers are becoming more astute in making health choices pertinent to their wellbeing, perhaps wanting also the practical help that is found within a therapeutic relationship, rather than just another prescription. This help may come in many guises, and the time spent within a caring relationship may be seen as central to the outcome of the reflexology treatment. Thus, an important question is whether this is the only reason for the dramatic relief from long-standing health problems frequently reported by some individuals following a course of reflexology. However, observations and interactions with clients suggest that there are other important outcomes from therapeutic encounters. It is also important to establish a platform of competence and trust, which values the judgement of clients and gives credence to their accounts of treatment and to use this to inform the evaluation of such treatment.

PRINCIPLES OF THE THERAPEUTIC RELATIONSHIP

Good reflexology practice is based on the following principles (adapted from Mitchell & Cormack 1998):

- The generation of a supportive therapeutic environment of openness and partnership conducive to self-awareness, growth and healing.
- A contract, which should be negotiated between the therapist and the client and which details the therapeutic process and potential outcomes, thus empowering the client to remain autonomous.
- Sound, relevant advice based on all available research evidence to facilitate the client's decision-making process, including consent to treatment or the opportunity to decline if they so wish.
- An individualized holistic approach to treatment with personal time for the client is made explicit as the philosophical and caring basis of the reflexology interaction.

- The therapist should work within the Professional Code(s) of Practice as the framework for safe effective practice, recognizing the boundaries as well as the potentials of reflexology.
- Adequate preparatory and continuing education, as well as mentor support and clinical supervision for ongoing practice.

CLIENT–THERAPIST INTERACTION

Everyday experience teaches us that good relationships are a recipe for harmony and progress, whereas bad relationships engender ill-will, pain and disharmony, and (taken to its extreme), destruction and death. Evidence to support this is seen in the many conflicts that continually take place at local, national and international levels. At every level of human society good relationships are applauded, thus indicating the high value accorded to them. From the moment of birth the child begins a long process of socialization, which is intended to make that individual appreciate and value relationships as an important aspect of good citizenship. It may therefore be said that the way we value relationships is steeped within our culture, and anything that affects their development can have a significant effect on the person's health–illness experience. Arnold & Boggs (1995) cite Piaget to emphasize the value of relationships and a nurturing environment in the development of children. It could therefore be argued that individuals brought up within a supportive, nurturing climate are likely to develop a more positive self-image as a basis for desirable relationships. However, the adverse effects of negative social and psychological experiences during key stages of development may result in problems in forming relationships later in life. For example, Stuart & Sundeem (1997) stress the importance of past events on present behaviour and Ingerman (1991) develops this further by suggesting that such negative experiences could result in the loss of part of the soul.

Relationships within the therapeutic environment can evoke a trusting bond between the client and the therapist, especially when they focus so deeply that it touches the essence of the person, in the attempt to generate healing energy. It may also be argued that the quality of the therapeutic relationship is more important than the actual therapy (Penson 1998). Mackereth (2000) suggests that being listened and attended to, combined with nurturing and holding touch, can be powerful, challenging and moving. The reflexologist must therefore be mindful of the way past events can impact on people's lives, and that individual experience may determine the state of readiness to enter into a (close) therapeutic relationship.

Positive and loving relationships are essential to all aspects of growth and development, and become even more essential to an individual who is experiencing health problems. Fundamental to the growth of the individual is personal autonomy, which imbues each person with certain unique characteristics of control, obligations, rights and responsibilities. This provides harmony in the person's life, enabling him or her to function as a relatively autonomous human being within society. Anything that poses a threat to that harmony will challenge their control, particularly ill health, and especially when the cause is unclear or the symptoms suggests a serious illness. Conversely, lack of harmony will affect the immune system and illness can occur. It is also thought that the mind, body and spirit are interconnected, a factor that takes account of the person's emotions, intellect, experience, values and beliefs, lifestyle and any other factor that makes the person unique (although Achterberg et al [1994 p 101] argue that this interconnection is the result of a chemical reaction within the body, such as of beta-endorphins). Reflexology focuses on this individual uniqueness and the concerns that each person brings to the therapeutic relationship, and can assist in returning the individual to a harmonious state, physically, emotionally and spiritually (Fig. 7.1, Plate 5).

The therapeutic encounter is a transforming process for the client (Wright & Sayre-Adams 2000), which is integrative, interactive and inseparable, thus holism is the cohesion of all matter (Davies 1997, Gerber 1988). Caring relationships should take place in a therapeutic environment that does not simply treat the physical problems but also creates a safe 'sacred

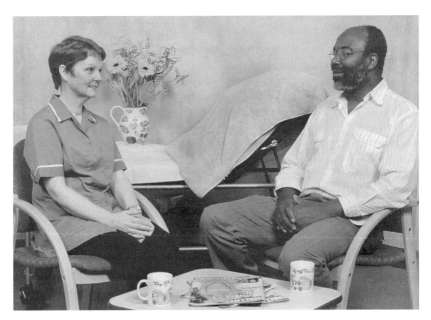

Figure 7.1 Establishing the client–patient relationship (see also Plate 5). Permissions from subjects of photo is hereby ackowledged.

space' (Wright & Sayre-Adams 2000) in which the holistic ideals can be met. The reflexologist can bring a range of qualities to the encounter that makes the environment conducive to healing, including clinical expertise, professionalism, compassion and an intention to heal. In this way the encounter becomes a positive healing experience, facilitating restoration of the energy balance to a point where the body's own healing potential can take over (Sayre-Adams & Wright 1995).

Touch can help to link people with their 'human-ness', helping them to share their feelings with others. Reflexology can unite two people in a therapeutic relationship through a process of interaction that benefits both, and, when the therapist displays unconditional regard and an image of positive feelings, the client will respond positively (Macrae 1988, Norman & Cowan 1998, Pitman & MacKenzie 1997, Sayre-Adams & Wright 1995). Robbins (1997) calls this a unity of purpose with therapeutic presence and suggests that 'it embodies the spatial and temporal characteristics of the therapeutic frame, and an experience of energy that may open, shut down, or disrupt the field of therapeutic contact'. Norman & Cowan (1998 p 22) report that the client and the therapist, on entering into this relationship 'feel grounded and can forget about the rest of the world' as the treatment takes place and that, through a process of sharing, varying degrees of satisfaction can be achieved that will form a good basis for initiating healing within the client.

This partnership is crucial to many aspects of care where the interaction is on a one-to-one basis, for example, counselling, psychotherapy, reflexology and other complementary therapies. These authors share the view of Pitman & MacKenzie (1997), who suggest that of the many skills and types of expertise used in reflexology, one of the most important is the establishment and development of the therapeutic relationship, reminding us of the uniqueness of each individual and the need to follow a holistic approach in working with each client. They cite the philosophy of Traditional Chinese Medicine in indicating the dynamic interplay of three sources of energy in the health–illness continuum: (i) the energy of the client; (ii) that of the practitioner; and (iii) the vital force.

MODELS FOR THERAPEUTIC RELATIONSHIPS

Holistic frameworks for care have been proposed by others (Tiran 1999) and can be adapted to facilitate an individualized approach to the care of reflexology clients. Using a model for clinical reflexology could facilitate the personal growth of the client and reflect the dynamic interactive process between the client and the reflexologist. In some cases a model may also provide an opportunity for personal growth and professional development of the practitioner. The purpose of the therapeutic relationship should be the empowerment and wellbeing of the client, set within the holistic model, which must take account of the many factors that can influence a person's existence, including psychosocial and economic circumstances, as well as health and disease. Whatever the cause and manifestations of ill health, it can result in loss of control, confidence and self-esteem, affecting the individual's capacity to meet daily needs. The therapist must therefore seek to establish a partnership that aims to raise the client's self-awareness, enabling the client to regain the locus of control, thus facilitating greater independence.

Interaction between the client and reflexologist is a complex phenomenon, influenced by a range of life events and experiences that can affect the relationship positively or negatively. These factors can inform the model for care and can be used to elicit a foundation within which the therapeutic relationship can thrive. The client and therapist may have different expectations of the treatment. The client, for example, may expect a 'cure' from an illness that so far has not responded to conventional medical treatment. Conversely, the therapist may wish to facilitate a situation in which the client can make lifestyle changes and decisions that will influence health and wellbeing. Good communication within an atmosphere of trust can help to develop a shared understanding of the proposed outcomes of treatment. It is frequently claimed that there are differences in the relationships between complementary therapist/client and orthodox practitioner/client. Sharma (1992) suggests that, in orthodox medicine, patients do not have many choices about their treatment, the responsibility often being handed over to the doctor. However, in choosing a complementary therapy such as reflexology, patients are exercising their right to make decisions about their own health care and are actively encouraged by their therapists to take this responsibility. Montbriand (1998) agrees with this idea and identifies the rekindling of hope as an important factor in the healing process. A therapeutic model for reflexology practice requires a contract between the client and therapist to facilitate and support this process.

Mantle (2001) argues that a model for practice can assist the therapist in making clinical judgements and Marks-Maran (1995) suggests that a model is a tool, which guides practice and facilitates reflection through which practice can be adapted and improved. Models of care are many and diverse but some have been adopted by healthcare professionals, such as nurses and counsellors, in order to enhance their practice (Reynolds & Cormack 1990). For example, Hume's behaviour therapy model focuses on factors such as lifestyle changes, stress management and assertiveness training in order to achieve personal growth; whereas Barker's cognitive therapy model is concerned with 'the intrinsic value of man' and assists people to revise their concept of themselves and the world around them to eliminate restrictive influences. Peplau uses an interpersonal relations model in nursing to empower patients through greater communication;

this is also reflected in Orem's self-care model. Smoyak's systems model emphasizes the interrelationship between the whole and the parts, each of which influence each other, whereas Roy's adaptation model focuses on the place of intervention and the need for adaptation in order to return to homeostasis. Rogers' (1983 p 284) client-centred model, essentially used in counselling, is based on the belief that human beings have the capacity to move from a state of psychological maladjustment to one of adjustment and suggests that a climate of mutual trust can promote personal growth and behavioural changes.

In summary, it can be seen that there are several common themes in these models, which can readily be applied to a philosophy for reflexology practice:

- lifestyle changes, particularly stress management
- revision of concept of self and environment
- empowerment through communication
- facilitation of self-care
- interrelationship between the whole and the parts
- need for intervention
- mutual trust.

A MODEL FOR REFLEXOLOGY PRACTICE

The model proposed here adopts an eclectic approach by integrating relevant aspects of other models, while taking into account the theories, principles and practice of reflexology. Our model for reflexology has four stages:

- Stage one – initial contact and dialogue
- Stage two – consultation and contract
- Stage three – therapeutic intervention
- Stage four – evaluation.

Stage one – the initial contact and dialogue

It is during this stage that rapport will be established between client and therapist. Information about the therapy can be given, together with a brief profile of the therapist's training and experience, which should help to reduce any initial anxiety the client may be feeling about the therapy. This first contact may be by telephone but the beginnings of a relationship can be facilitated by a sensitive attitude and providing information in an easy-to-understand manner. It is important to establish whether or not reflexology can be of benefit to this client and whether the reflexologist is able to meet the client's needs before proceeding to Stage two. Practitioners must acknowledge their personal parameters and decline to step beyond the boundaries of their professional competence and experience (see Chapter 4).

Stage two – consultation and contract (assessment and planning)

Clients visit a reflexologist for a variety of physical, psychological and emotional health issues. Whatever the reason for the consultation, there may be a degree of anticipatory anxiety, for example, concern about whether the treatment will work or be harmful, or simply worrying about trying something that is not part of orthodox medicine. Professional reflexologists should endeavour to put their clients at ease at the first consultation, and to inform them about the potential value of the therapeutic intervention. Relevant biographical data and a full medical history should be taken and the basis of the client–therapist relationship should be outlined, followed by a detailed explanation of the intended reflexology treatment, including the potential benefits, possible side-effects and reactions. It is also at this point that the reflexologist and client should agree a working contract, which clearly sets out their respective rights, obligations and boundaries, as well as the flexibility to renegotiate, should there be changes in the client's condition or circumstances (see Chapters 4 and 9). Every client should be treated as an individual and factors such as the length of contract and the need to review the outcome of treatment to assess the benefits will be different for each client. Clients need to be assured that confidential records are maintained and that no other person will be informed about the condition of the client unless permission has been granted. Within the contract, a 24-hour notice of cancellation may be agreed for subsequent appointments. It should also be made clear that the client can withdraw at any point if there is dissatisfaction or unease with any aspect of treatment. The contract should be agreed in such a way that it demonstrates respect and value for the individual and an ethos of mutual trust should be established as a basis for the quality of communication that should be expected, as this informs the whole treatment process. Clients must trust that the reflexologist will work in their best interests and respond sympathetically to stated needs, whilst practitioners must trust clients to work in partnership with them (Box 7.1). As the relationship develops the level of trust will grow and the individual client should feel more relaxed at subsequent consultations. Mackereth (2000) suggests that the therapist should be focused, with the client at the centre of the therapeutic interaction at all times, as it is important to be aware of the verbal and non-verbal cues given by the client.

Stage three – the therapeutic intervention (implementation)

It is during this stage that the real channels of communication should begin to open up between the client and reflexologist, although the pace

---

Box 7.1   Reflexology in partnership

Fiona saw her midwife–reflexologist in the complementary therapy antenatal clinic when she was 26 weeks pregnant, having been referred for frequent and severe panic attacks. She was extremely talkative and appeared very anxious, although this did not seem to be directly related to the pregnancy. Every time the reflexologist tried to answer a question or give some advice Fiona attempted to 'talk over' her. Fiona had been prescribed medication by her GP to deal with the panic attacks but she had declined to take it, in the mistaken belief that it was unsafe to do so. She had, however, chosen to listen to the (incorrect) advice of her sister regarding the use of aromatherapy essential oils and was using these with no effect and some unrecognized risk to herself and the baby. The practitioner suggested that reflexology, combined with some of the Bach flower remedies, might be helpful. However, the practitioner needed three attempts before Fiona would listen to her sufficiently to assure her that she had understood. The reflexologist explained that she would expect Fiona to make a choice about her treatment: she could decline to return if she so wished, but if she intended to continue with the treatment it was important that she work in partnership with the reflexologist. Advice and treatment given would be based on all available evidence as to its relevance to pregnancy, safety and efficacy and Fiona would not be asked to have inappropriate treatments. However, Fiona would need to agree to fulfil her side of the contract in order for the treatment to be given a chance to work. Fiona agreed to 'give it a go' but, sadly, did not return for her second appointment.

---

and extent to which this occurs will vary with each individual, as some relationships develop more readily than others. Every effort should be made to maintain an open and supportive environment, to reduce anxiety, generate a climate of trust and facilitate the client to share genuine health concerns with the reflexologist. This may include previous experience and evaluation of conventional or complementary treatment. The practice of 'greeting the feet' (Pitman & MacKenzie 1997) should be given high priority by the clinical reflexologist for holding the feet in a caring way conveys to the client the clear desire to help and heal. It is at this point that the therapeutic relationship truly begins and the reflexologist begins to work with the client on many levels with the purpose of initiating healing. Communication should be two-way and will be explicit and implicit, verbal and non-verbal, biophysical, psychoemotional and may be in the form of energy transfer between therapist and client.

A competent reflexologist will aim to keep things in perspective in terms of what reflexology has to offer, without either over- or underestimating its benefits or limitations. An example of this is the relaxed state that most people feel or the 'healing crisis' experienced by some clients (see Chapter 6). Treatment should be adapted according to the client's reactions and responses at the time. Advisably, a contact number should be given to any client who may be concerned about potential post-treatment reactions. Some clients may also be taught simple techniques that they might find useful between treatments.

Stage four – evaluation

This is the final phase in the treatment event and is where the reflexologist invites questions and comments from the client to address issues that may not have been dealt with earlier in the interactions. These should be dealt with clearly and honestly, and in as much detail as the client requires and is able to assimilate at this point. It is also important to consider issues of safety in reflexology treatment, for example, ensuring the client is sufficiently alert after a short rest to make the return journey home safely. The treatment session should close with the knowledge and satisfaction that the client has received the highest standard of care.

CONCLUSION

It could be argued that the time spent with a client is the most important part of the reflexology treatment, although a valuable therapeutic relationship is achievable even when time is limited because it is the interaction between client and therapist that assists in the perception of overall wellbeing of the client. On the other hand, there is some evidence to suggest that reflexology can be effective as a treatment for specific conditions, irrespective of the relationship between client and therapist or the time they spend together.

The therapeutic relationship is an encounter to which clients and therapists bring their own values, beliefs and prejudices, which affect the quality of the interaction and, ultimately, the entire healing process for the individual. By using a model for the therapeutic interaction, reflexologists can focus more effectively on establishing rapport with clients, thereby creating an environment in which a high standard of holistic care can be generated. This can empower clients to regain and retain control over their own health and wellbeing. Using a contract within such a framework secures an environment of trust and care that enables clients to make choices, leading to positive self-regard. This should enhance the healing potential of the reflexology treatment, resulting in a positive outcome for both parties.

In considering the importance of communication within a caring therapeutic relationship Davis & Fallowfield (1991) cite Kierkegaard, who suggests that in order to help someone the carer should first seek to understand the client. It is also important that the reflexologist ensures that the client understands the potential benefits of reflexology. Accordingly, if the reflexologist practises within the framework of the model and principles outlined within this chapter, the therapeutic relationship should make a significant contribution towards the practice of reflexology.

REFERENCES

Achterberg J, Dossey B, Kolkmeier L. Rituals of healing: using imagery for health and wellness. London: Bantam Books; 1994.

Arnold E, Boggs K. Professional interpersonal relationships: communication skills for nurses. London: WB Saunders; 1995.

Chard J, Lilford RJ, Gardner D. Looking beyond the next patient: sociology and modern health care. Lancet 1999; 353(9151):486–489.

Davies CM. Complementary therapies in rehabilitation: holistic approaches for prevention and wellness. London: Slack Incorporated; 1997.

Davis H, Fallowfield L. Counselling and communication in health care. Chichester: John Wiley & Sons; 1991.

Gerber R. Vibrational medicine. Santa Fe, CA: Bear and Company; 1988.

Hill J. ed. Rheumatology nursing: a creative approach. London: Churchill Livingstone; 1998.

Ingerman S. Soul retrieval: mending the fragmented self. San Francisco, CA: Harper; 1991.

Khan M. Between therapist and client: the new relationship. New York: WH Freeman and Company; 1997.

Liossi C, Mystakidou K. Heron's theory of human needs in palliative care. European Journal of Palliative Care 1997; 4(1):32–35.

Mackereth P. Tough places to be tender: contracting for happy or "good enough" endings in therapeutic massage/bodywork? Complementary Therapies in Nursing and Midwifery 2000; 6(3):111–115.

Macrae J. Therapeutic touch: a practical guide. London: Penguin; 1988.

Mantle F. Complementary therapies and nursing models. In: Rankin-Box D, ed. The Nurses' Handbook of Complementary Therapies. 2nd edn. London: Baillière Tindall; 2001:63–72.

Marchione J. Margaret Newman: health as expanding consciousness. London: Sage Publications; 1993.

Marks-Maran D. Procrustes in the ward: fitting people into models. In: Jolley M, Bryczynska G, eds. Nursing beyond tradition and conflict. London: Mosby; 1995.

Mitchell A, Cormack M. The therapeutic relationship in complementary health care. London: Churchill Livingstone; 1998.

Montbriand MJ. Abandoning biomedicine for alternative therapies: oncology patients' stories. Cancer Nursing 1998; 21(1):36–45.

Norman L, Cowan T. The reflexology handbook: a complete guide. London: Piatkus; 1998.

Pitman V, MacKenzie K. Reflexology: a practical approach. Cheltenham: Stanley Thornes Publishers; 1997.

Penson J. Complementary therapies: making a difference in palliative care. Complementary Therapies in Nursing and Midwifery 1998; 4(3):77–81.

Reynolds W, Cormack D, eds. Psychiatric and mental health nursing: theory and practice. London: Chapman and Hall; 1990.

Robbins A ed. Therapeutic presence bridging expression and form. London: Jessica Kingsley Publishers; 1997. Available: http://www.jkp.com/catalogue/inter/rob_the.html

Rogers C. Freedom to learn for the 80's. Columbus, OH: Merrill Publishing Company; 1983.

Sayre-Adams J, Wright SG. The theory and practice of therapeutic touch. London: Churchill Livingstone; 1995.

Sharma U. Complementary medicine today. Practitioners and patients. London: Tavistock/Routledge; 1992.

Stuart GW, Sundeem MT. Principles and practice of psychiatric nursing. London: Mosby; 1997.

Tiran D. A holistic framework for maternity care. Complementary Therapies in Nursing and Midwifery 1999; 5(5):127–135.

Wright SG, Sayre-Adams J. Sacred space: right relationships and spirituality in healthcare. London: Churchill Livingstone; 2000.

8

Practising safely and effectively: introducing the 'No Hands' approach, a paradigm shift in the theory and practice of reflexology

Gerry Pyves and Peter A Mackereth

Traditional recommendations for the practice of reflexology	Postural principles
	Techniques
Taking care of the practitioner	**Conclusion**
Introducing the theories and principles of 'No Hands' reflexology	**References**

The following material is drawn from the work of Gerry Pyves, the originator of 'No Hands' massage, and is amended from his forthcoming book entitled 'The theory and practice of No Hands reflexology'.

Editors' note. The Editors feel that this innovative and original work is worthy of inclusion in a text on clinical reflexology at a time when there is increasing recognition of the risk element of clinical practice, in all areas of health care, both for clients and for practitioners. The work challenges some traditional approaches to reflexology and has arisen through personal experience, observation of traditional bodywork techniques and a recent survey commissioned by the author (Watson 2000). It is important to emphasize that research work is needed formally to evaluate this and other

Abstract

The work of Pyves with practitioners of massage and other forms of bodywork is well documented (Pyves 2000, 2001a, b, c). He started working without using the hands in the early 1980s, after sustaining a personal wrist injury. Full-time clinical work became impossible using conventional massage techniques and the 'No Hands' system of massage was developed as an alternative means of performing a variety of forms of bodywork techniques.

The primary aim of 'No Hands' reflexology is to enable practitioners to work reflex points in the client without using their own hands or fingers. This chapter explores the concept of performing reflexology in this way to avoid injury to the therapist and re-evaluates conventional reflexology techniques. The chapter also briefly identifies and discusses other key issues related to the practice of clinical reflexology (some of which are explored more fully in other chapters).

approaches to bodywork to provide evidence to inform safe and effective practice. Readers are asked to read this chapter in good faith and to use it as an opportunity critically to review traditional patterns of working in reflexology.

Key words: injury, 'No Hands', safety

It is over 200 years since Per Henrik Ling's Swedish 'movement cure' was developed with the well-known classification of different massage strokes, including effleurage, petrissage, friction, vibration and tapotement (Benjamin 1993, Goldstone 2000), yet there does not appear to have been an evaluation of, or challenge to, the basic rationale for Ling's massage techniques being performed exclusively with the hands (Tappan 1988).

In reflexology there is a high risk of injury to the hands and wrists from constantly using the thumbs and fingers. For example, this can be seen in the repetitive nature of the traditional 'caterpillar crawling' movement. In an exploratory study commissioned by Gerry Pyves, a comprehensive questionnaire of 350 randomly selected massage practitioners to assess the extent of injury as a result of their practice (Watson 2000) over 78% reported injury to their hands and wrists alone, with some having related injury or trauma, for example, to the spine. This supported the earlier findings of Greene (1995). Pyves and others have observed that injury appears to develop over seven clearly defined stages, (Fig. 8.1), but is often not recognized by the individual until the injury has reached Stage 4 (Adams, cited in Pyves 2000). This suggests that the incidence of injury could be higher than 78%, an alarming figure for a relatively small profession.

TRADITIONAL RECOMMENDATIONS FOR THE PRACTICE OF REFLEXOLOGY

As with many helping professions, the focus is usually on how best to deliver the intervention to patients, and not always on the impact this might have on the practitioner over time. Safe working practices have evolved (often as a result of legal claims for work related injury, subjected to the burden of proof). The difficulty with reflexology and other bodywork practices is that this is often too late, given that it may have happened over years, and in private practice, where there is no employer to seek recompense from. Where reflexologists are working as employees there may not as yet be policies and training for reflexology-specific health and safety guidelines. Reflexologists are therefore often purely reliant on what they have learnt from the training and the reflexology literature.

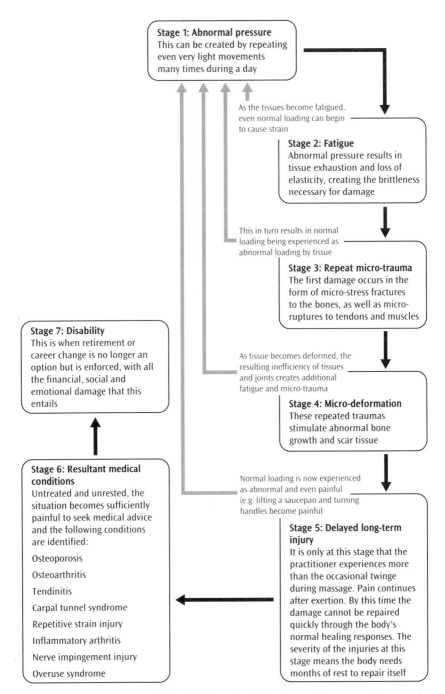

Stage 1: Abnormal pressure
This can be created by repeating even very light movements many times during a day

As the tissues become fatigued, even normal loading can begin to cause strain

Stage 2: Fatigue
Abnormal pressure results in tissue exhaustion and loss of elasticity, creating the brittleness necessary for damage

This in turn results in normal loading being experienced as abnormal loading by tissue

Stage 3: Repeat micro-trauma
The first damage occurs in the form of micro-stress fractures to the bones, as well as micro-ruptures to tendons and muscles

Stage 7: Disability
This is when retirement or career change is no longer an option but is enforced, with all the financial, social and emotional damage that this entails

As tissue becomes deformed, the resulting inefficiency of tissues and joints creates additional fatigue and micro-trauma

Stage 4: Micro-deformation
These repeated traumas stimulate abnormal bone growth and scar tissue

Stage 6: Resultant medical conditions
Untreated and unrested, the situation becomes sufficiently painful to seek medical advice and the following conditions are identified:

Osteoporosis

Osteoarthritis

Tendinitis

Carpal tunnel syndrome

Repetitive strain injury

Inflammatory arthritis

Nerve impingement injury

Overuse syndrome

Normal loading is now experienced as abnormal and even painful (e.g. lifting a saucepan and turning handles become painful

Stage 5: Delayed long-term injury
It is only at this stage that the practitioner experiences more than the occasional twinge during massage. Pain continues after exertion. By this time the damage cannot be repaired quickly through the body's normal healing responses. The severity of the injuries at this stage means the body needs months of rest to repair itself

Figure 8.1   The seven stages of injury. The key point is that the practitioner experiences serious pain only at Stage 5, occasional twinges at Stage 4 and no pain before this (from Pyves 2001c).

The typical position for giving a reflexology treatment is sedentary, with the practitioner facing the patient and 'application of the technique by the human hand to the human foot' (Kunz & Kunz 1993 p 154). While advantageous in terms of visually observing and interacting with the patient, this 'constant attentiveness' (Dougans 1995 p 82) can limit physical activity and opportunities to relax and flow in the work. Recommendations have been made to build up a good sitting position; Lett (2000) states 'an erect, supple posture is graceful and attractive' (p 95) and suggests that the practitioner 'makes it part of her practice to sit well . . . feet place firmly on the floor . . . avoid slumping . . . the head should remain erect' (p. 96). Although this is good advice if a practitioner is limited to one posture, what is missing is discussion on ways of working effectively, without strain or discomfort. If practitioners can work comfortably, and even in a way that benefits their own health, this must in turn improve the quality of attention and touch given to the patients.

Using instruments to replace the human hand is not recommended in this book or by other leading authors (Kunz & Kunz 1993, Lett 2000, Marquardt 2000) because they create a barrier between the patient and practitioner and are incapable of sensing resistance, assessing temperature and palpating the condition of the tissues and underlying muscle. Lett (2000) suggests some ways of working with the hands and maintaining contact with the patient (Box 8.1).

These points are claimed to be helpful in maintaining safe and effective working with the hands, and emphasize that reflexology is not purely about exerting pressure on areas of the feet. However, it is important to recognize that not all reflexologists work on one foot and then another, thus requiring covering of the untended foot. It is possible to work between the feet, comparing and contrasting areas and responses to palpation. Either way, the most important aspect is keeping the room warm for the comfort of both the patient and practitioner. Keeping contact with the patient also does not require continuous skin-to-skin contact. There are other ways of remaining in contact, for example, working over towels, including eye and verbal contact, and in some situations incorporating 'off the body' work. Later in this chapter some innovative approaches are suggested, which take the work beyond hand contact.

Box 8.1 The basic treatment movement (Lett 2000 pp 96–97)

1. Movements made by thumbs or fingers should always be directed away from the body.
2. Effective treatment is not about exerting pressure but probing and feeling the 'give'.
3. All treatments should be rhythmical, flowing and without hesitation – 'wave-like'.
4. One hand should remain in contact with the feet at all times – unbroken contact.
5. When working on one foot only, the other foot should be kept amply and warmly covered.

TAKING CARE OF THE PRACTITIONER

As with other professions engaged in therapeutic work, practitioners are drawn to their work because they want to help others. Parkin (2000) acknowledges this common intention in suggesting that reflexologists are often natural 'givers' and because of that 'or through ignorance or neglect, may put their own health and body at risk' (Parkin 2000 p 27). Dougans (1995) argues that reflexologists should be an 'asset' to reflexology, acting as healthy role models, abiding by their own health advice and presenting a healthy image (Dougans 1995 p 82). Training may include some mention of safe working practices, but this often focuses on hygiene concerns and learning traditional working practices, such as using the hands and being seated for giving treatments. In clinical practice with patients who are in bed or sitting in low chairs, finding ways of adapting treatments is crucial (see Section 2).

Physical comfort is not the only issue facing practitioners, for example, personal safety is increasingly a concern for therapists in a variety of settings (Box 8.2). Parkin (2000) raises concerns about the risks of working alone as a woman and being potentially at risk from some male clients. It is important to assess potential clients carefully, to consider working in a shared space and, if there is any fear about working with an individual, to decide not to treat them. Importantly, there are ways of examining and developing working practices that protect both the practitioner and client, such as clinical supervision (see Chapter 2). Practitioners can also obtain support by participating in a peer support group or a reflexology organization, as well as engaging in strategies for maintaining personal health and wellbeing (see Chapter 6).

The new approach of 'No Hands' requires a rethink of every aspect of the reflexologist's own movements and encourages the work to be seen as a form of mediation or Tai Chi (Pyves 2001c). It shifts the focus to the shared space and interaction in which the benefits are reciprocal. The act of giving and receiving reflexology then becomes a truly shared experience. Feeling

---

Box 8.2   Examples of working and safety problems

- Abuse from patients – verbal, physical, sexual and psychological.
- Acute and/or enduring physical injury/damage from poor working practices.
- Overworking and burnout – anxiety, changes in body weight, sleep problems, headaches, etc.
- Adopting unhelpful coping behaviours to deal with work-related stress – overeating, substance abuse, working in a mechanistic manner, etc.
- Reduced work performance – loss of clients, money, interprofessional difficulties.
- Legal and ethical issues – confidentiality concerns when a patient discloses information that is relevant to the safety of others or to the patient personally, e.g. suicidal thoughts (see Chapter 4).

good after giving reflexology is no longer an afterthought or an occasional reflection, but a central tenet of the work. This reframing and re-evaluation of how we practise as reflexologists creates and celebrates healing synergy – where reflexologist and patient are no longer the healer and the healee, but share in the process of healing.

INTRODUCING THE THEORIES AND PRINCIPLES OF 'NO HANDS' REFLEXOLOGY

There are many philosophies and approaches to reflexology, many based on traditional Indian or Chinese medicine. In modern reflexology, Ingham built on ancient theories (Ingham 1984) and Arnold (2000) also links practice to oriental bodywork. Pyves (2001b) believes that it is not necessary for each therapy to be isolationist in its practice and that it is acceptable for elements of other therapies to be incorporated, for example, some Swedish massage strokes can feasibly be utilized when performing reflexology. Indeed, Pyves acknowledges that most bodywork practitioners will stimulate many of the reflex points on the bodies of their clients, and suggests that reflexology as a discrete therapy does not hold a monopoly on ownership of these reflex points. Acupressure, Thai massage, shiatsu and triggerpoint work in structural massage all utilize knowledge of reflex points within their practices.

Pyves believes that the reflexes are situated in the body between the bone and the muscle, although he accepts that he has no evidence of this theory. In areas where muscles are tight, it may be impossible to stimulate the reflexes deep beneath, despite any attempts to do so, for the muscle acts as a form of protection of the reflexes. However, neurological impulses have initiated the muscle tension and indirect relaxation should occur as a result of psychologically relaxing the client. For this reason, the preparatory work on the soft tissues could be said to be almost more important than the stimulation of the reflexes, a process which will facilitate the client's own innate healing potential to self-stimulate the reflexes.

POSTURAL PRINCIPLES

This, then, appears to contradict the traditional method of applying reflexology techniques by precise and minute stimulation of pinhead-sized reflex points on the feet, and lends weight to a possible argument for a more diffuse manipulation, stimulation and massage of the feet, whilst continuing to produce a therapeutic effect by working on the reflex points indirectly. By 'opening up' the soft tissues through deep and powerful movements, the reflexes are stimulated with less effort and more effect.

'No Hands' reflexology assists in achieving this widespread reflex stimulation and the impact of close physical contact between the client and the practitioner continues to produce a therapeutically nurturing effect. 'No Hands' reflexology practitioners use the forearms and their own feet in a way not dissimilar to shiatsu techniques.

To adapt reflexology practice to this method, seven postural principles need to be considered for safe and effective practice. They are based on the oriental philosophies from which many Eastern therapies draw theory and practice.

1. *Hara* is the source of energy within practitioners that enables them to perform effectively. This energy is thought to originate from the abdomen of the therapist, and is the centre from which all meridians (energy lines) emanate outwards to and from the limbs. *Hara* is considered to be the source of life force and nourishment whilst in the uterus and is the place into which we inhale and from which we exhale.

2. *Sole* is the process of 'grounding' often referred to in bodywork, and results from a 'dropping down' of the practitioner's bodyweight into the feet and knees. This provides an anchoring which empowers the reflexology (or other bodywork) movements.

3. *Flow* involves the dynamic image of the water element and the concept of 'whole body flow'; the practitioner becomes this constantly moving medium. This elemental approach enhances variety in the reflexology or massage session, enabling an ebb and flow of rhythm and pace. This principle also avoids the stiffening of posture and the locked rigidity often seen in practitioners attempting to maintain 'proper' posture. Pyves, like Feldenkrais (1977), eschews the very concept of 'good' posture, for a dynamic concept of movement and balance. The psychological impact on therapists will result in a physiological effect to protect them from any pathological injury. In other words, if therapists are mentally relaxed and flowing, the body will remain relaxed, thereby avoiding those muscle tensions that lead to postural rigidity and the risk of injury.

4. *Falling* is a fundamental component of 'No Hands' reflexology in which the practitioner almost literally 'falls' onto the client, although this should more correctly be thought of as a leaning onto rather than a pushing against the client. Leaning provides counterpressure, enabling a slow transference of bodyweight whilst creating a powerful and sensitive pressure. This also ensures that the bodyweight of the therapist is distributed in varying proportions onto the feet and hands. However, it might be necessary to adjust the height of the couch to achieve a solid foundation for the practitioner and to alter the traditional posture, in which it is primarily the hands, shoulders and upper body of the therapist that take any strain caused by poor posture.

5. *Kneeling* to perform some of the reflexology session facilitates some powerful therapeutic strokes yet ensures that the practitioner maintains

good posture, keeping the back straight and allowing the lower body to manoeuvre. Again, adjustment of the couch may be necessary.

6. *Support* involves utilizing the various stabilizing surfaces around the practitioner including the table struts and the client's own body, to ensure correct posture.

7. *Shire* refers to the principle of always employing a vastly superior weight : force ratio in the practitioner to effect therapeutic pressure on the client. This is very relevant in the preparatory work of warming, loosening, stretching and kneading the soft tissues of the client prior to stimulating the reflexes beneath, in much the same way as a shire horse pulls a plough to loosen the ground before seed can be sowed. If the 'ploughing' is performed effectively there may be no real need to stimulate the reflexes directly as they will have surfaced naturally and been facilitated to self-heal.

TECHNIQUES

'No Hands' massage, utilizing the seven postural principles, produces systemic effects on the client without risk of injury to the practitioner. Softer and larger parts of the practitioner's body are used to apply therapeutic power without pain or discomfort for the client. This avoids the limitations on professional practice that conventional thumb and finger work might have in the event of sustaining an injury.

Pyves (2000) has identified 23 points of the therapist's body that can be used to apply pressure to the client. Although it is not possible here to discuss all 23, Fig. 8.2 shows the array of different surfaces that can be used on the forearm alone, and two of the 70 new techniques of 'No Hands' reflexology, the 'foot mangle' and the 'reflexor' are described below.

The 'foot mangle'

Figure 8.3 (Plate 6) demonstrates the 'foot mangle' technique with the client lying prone. The 'foot mangle' is performed with the client's ankle positioned in the anterior angle of the practitioner's forearm, using the other arm to massage the sole of the foot. In addition, the therapist leans away from the client's hips, thus creating a simultaneous stretch on the Achilles tendon by pushing the ball of the foot towards the couch. The practitioner may be standing, crouching or kneeling and facing in a variety of directions. Deep muscle tension release occurs in the whole foot and leg, creating a 'mangle' effect and replacing numerous different massage strokes, yet having effects similar to effleurage and petrissage. If the practitioner also transfers bodyweight alternately towards and away from the client's hips and spine, a rhythmic, hypnotic, relaxing movement is achieved, which has a systemic effect on the client, opening up the reflex channels to work distally on the relevant body parts and organs. Very deep massage can be

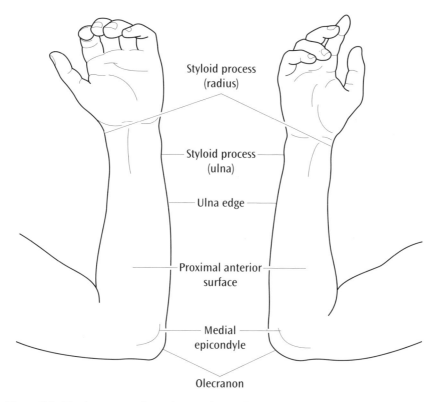

Figure 8.2   The foream – surfaces that can be used to apply pressure (from Pyves 2001c).

applied to the plantar surface of the foot by laying the foot on the couch with the practitioner leaning the whole of the upper bodyweight onto the client. Pressure is removed by the practitioner straightening the torso and lifting the working forearm off the client's foot.

Figure 8.4 (Plate 7) demonstrates the 'foot mangle' technique with the client lying supine. In this position, the technique works on the plantar and dorsal surfaces of the client's foot. It requires the practitioner to kneel at 45° to the client with contact on both foot surfaces, creating the 'mangle' effect, which can replace effleurage.

The 'reflexor'

Figure 8.5 (Plate 8) demonstrates the 'reflexor' technique with the client lying prone. The 'reflexor' involves using the soft surface of the arm to work on the client's sole and the olecranon to stimulate specific reflexes. The non-working hand can be placed underneath the client's foot enabling the

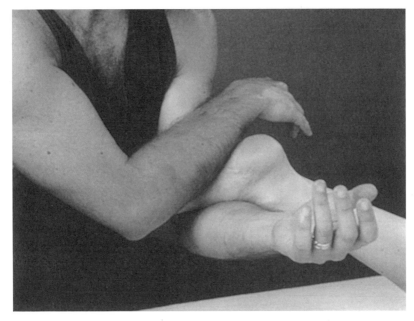

Figure 8.3   The 'foot mangle' technique. The client is lying prone (see also Plate 6).

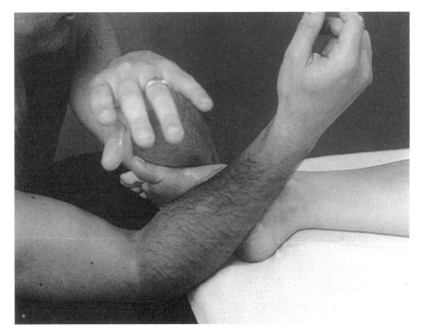

Figure 8.4   The 'foot mangle' technique. The client is lying supine (see also Plate 7).

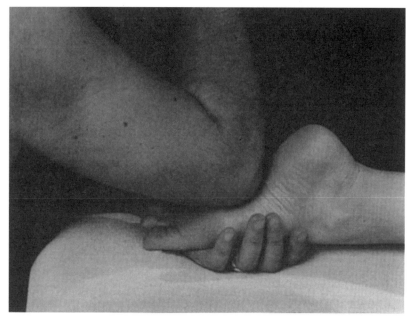

Figure 8.5 The 'reflexor' technique. The client is lying prone (see also Plate 8).

practitioner to be responsive to the foot anatomy and to the nuances of minor responses from the client. Different movements of the body and arm will create a variety of reflex stimulations ranging from subtle vibrational techniques to more direct and forceful approaches. The technique enables the practitioner to work all the reflex points on the toes, sole and heel, as well as many of the spinal points on the medial surface of the foot. Deep yet gentle relaxation can be achieved which may enhance the therapeutic relationship.

Figure 8.6 (Plate 9) demonstrates the 'reflexor' technique with the client lying supine. The practitioner maintains a secure and supported position and then by turning the foot slightly outwards and supporting it with the resting hand, reflexes on the sole and medial surface of the foot can be worked.

CONCLUSION

As a consequence of developing new techniques that could protect therapists from hand and wrist injury, Pyves discovered that his reflexology practice became more powerful and effective and surmises that by opening up the reflex areas with this soothing, deep and gentle massage, conventional reflexology techniques become almost redundant. The 'No Hands' reflexology system can be used irrespective of the practitioner's individual philosophy. In

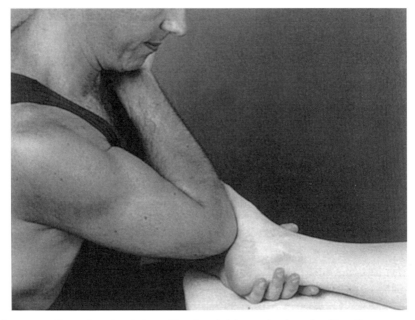

Figure 8.6 The 'reflexor' technique. The client is lying supine (see also Plate 9).

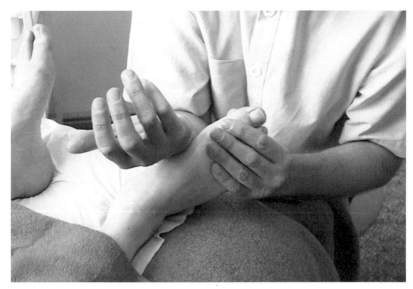

Figure 8.7 Another illustration of using a surface of the forearm for reflexology (see also Plate 10). Photo courtesy of Katie Spruce BA (Hons), medical photographer, Christie Hospital NHS Trust, with permission.

more scientific theory, the technique, in effect, uses Newtonian principles, in which any force (on the client's foot) produces an equal and opposite force (on the practitioner's hands). Similarly, sheer appreciation of the anatomical variations in strength between the wrist, with its complex structure of numerous bones, and the more robust long bones of the forearm imply that there is a value in adapting the techniques of conventional reflexology to reduce the risk of practitioner injury. This should now be investigated in a more formal way in order to demonstrate its effectiveness and safety – it could become the 'new reflexology' practice for all therapists.

This chapter has suggested a new approach to working. It is also important to acknowledge that there are other issues, briefly discussed in this chapter and elsewhere in this book, relevant to working safely and effectively. The 'No Hands' approach is suggested as a means of taking care of ourselves in practice as reflexologists (Fig. 8.7, Plate 10). In doing so we honour being an important part of healing synergy, which in turns benefits our patients.

REFERENCES

Adams A. Degenerative masseur's syndrome. Workshop presentation. Cited in Pyves G. The principles and practice of 'No Hands' massage – zero strain bodywork. Huddersfield: Shi'Zen Publications; 2000.
Arnold MM. Chi-reflexology: guidelines for the middle way. Australia: Moss M Arnold Publications; 2000.
Benjamin P. Massage therapy in the 1940s and the College of Swedish Massage in Chicago. Massage Therapy Journal 1993; 32(4):56.
Dougans I. The art of reflexology. Dorset: Element Books; 1995.
Greene L. Save your hands. Florida: Gilded Age Press; 1995.
Feldenkrais M. Awareness through movement: health exercise for personal growth. New York: Penguin; 1977.
Goldstone LA. Massage as an orthodox medical treatment past and future. Complementary Therapies in Nursing and Midwifery 2000; 6(4):169–175.
Ingham E. The original works of Eunice D Ingham: stories the feet can tell thru reflexology and stories the feet have told thru reflexology. St Petersburg, FL: Ingham Publishing, Inc; 1984.
Kunz K, Kunz B. The complete guide to foot reflexology (revised). Albuquerque, New Mexico: Reflexology Research; 1993.
Lett A. Reflex zone therapy for health professionals. London: Churchill Livingstone; 2000.
Marquardt H. Reflexotherapy of the feet. New York: Thieme; 2000.
Parkin E. Self-care for reflexologists. Reflexions: Journal of the Association of Reflexologists 2000; 60:27.
Pyves G. The principles and practice of 'No Hands' massage – zero strain bodywork. Huddersfield: Shi'Zen Publications; 2000.
Pyves G. Injurious massage techniques – silence of the lambs. Holistic Therapist 2001a; 8:19–21.
Pyves G. Massage history – from technique to therapy. Holistic Therapist 2001b; 9:19–22.
Pyves G. 'No Hands' massage – squaring the circle of practitioner damage. Journal of Bodywork and Movement Therapies 2001c; 5(3):173–180.
Tappan FM. Healing massage techniques: holistic, classic and emerging methods. 2nd edn. Northwalk, CT: Appleton and Lange; 1988.
Watson D. An investigation into the links between massage practice and musculoskeletal damage to the practitioner's hands and wrists. Huddersfield: Shi'Zen Publications; 2000.

Application of reflexology in specialist clinical areas

Introduction

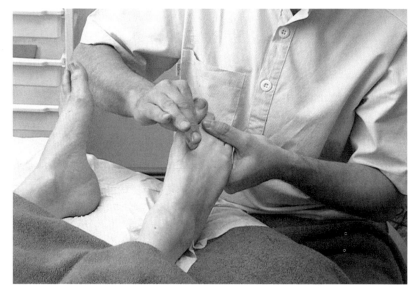

Photo courtesy of Katie Spruce BA (Hons), medical photographer, Christie Hospital NHS Trust, with permission.

Section 1 explored contemporary themes related to the clinical practice of reflexology. Section 2 focuses on the professional practice issues relevant to integrating reflexology within specified clinical areas. The contributing authors bring to each of the six chapters their specialized experience and expertise of using reflexology in the areas chosen. The list of practice arenas is not exhaustive, rather, this section presents exemplars of innovative work by reflexologists within the field of health care.

The authors consider the issues and concerns that need to be addressed when integrating reflexology. Reflective accounts, case study material and the available literature are utilized to raise and explore important issues and, where possible, recommendations are made for best practice.

Chapter 9. Integrating reflexology in conventional healthcare settings by Peter Mackereth. The first chapter in this section is by way of an introduction to the processes and stages necessary for greater integration. The recommendations for best practice are based on the evaluation of a reflexology evaluation project, review of the literature and the author's experience of integrating and coordinating complementary therapy services in acute hospital care.

Chapter 10. Supporting women during pregnancy and childbirth by Denise Tiran. In this chapter, a practising complementary therapist and midwife explores the uses, safety, precautions and potential complications of using reflexology during pregnancy and childbirth. The legal implications for practitioners who are not qualified midwives are discussed, placing the emphasis firmly on professional accountability.

Chapter 11. Practising in the neonatal area by Liz Tipping. The author considers the value of practising reflexology in the neonatal environment. The fragile condition of preterm babies, while making it difficult to consider this intervention, has led the author instead to examine the benefits of reflexology for parents, especially the mother, with the focus on managing stress and facilitating lactation.

Chapter 12. Advocating the use of reflexology for people with a learning disability by Evelyn Gale. This chapter explores the value of reflexology for people with a learning disability, including its use within a Snoezelen environment. Other issues pertinent to the practice of reflexology specifically with this client group are also considered.

Chapter 13. Improving and maintaining mental health by Christine Knowles and Grace Higgins. The authors examine the use of reflexology as a therapeutic intervention for those experiencing mental health problems such as stress, anxiety and depression, which may compromise their ability to cope with the pace and change of modern life. They also consider issues of safety and protection for both client and practitioner.

Chapter 14. Enhancing quality of life for people in palliative care settings by Edwina Hodkinson and Julia Williams. This chapter examines the fears and myths that can emerge when offering reflexology to people who have cancer and other life-limiting illnesses, and suggests ways of adapting reflexology to meet specific needs and manage certain symptoms. Most importantly, the chapter debates key issues around the integration of clinical reflexology into conventional care for people in palliative care settings.

9

Integrating reflexology in conventional healthcare settings

Peter A Mackereth

Abstract

There is evidence of the growing use of reflexology in a number of areas of
healthcare practice, including maternity care, hospital daycare units, GP practices
and hospices. Surveys by Hayes & Cox (1999) and Rankin-Box (1997) have identified
that reflexology is now even being used in intensive care and coronary care units.
This chapter will explore some of the key issues in offering reflexology as an
integrated service, with an emphasis on acute hospital care. The recommendations
for best practice are based on the evaluation of a pilot reflexology project (Dryden et
al 1998, 1999; Cromwell et al 1999), review of the literature and the author's
experience of integrating and coordinating complementary therapy services.

**Key words: provision, protocols and policies, funding, audit,
supervision**

Surgical interventions and medical therapies continue to evolve and
offer hope to people with acute and chronic health problems. However,
both patients and healthcare staff acknowledge that technology and
aggressive treatments are not the only answers to providing care and improving wellbeing. Stone (2001 p 55) suggests that both in the UK and the US
there has been a significant shift towards 'integrated (or integrative)
health care' and greater tolerance towards the inclusion of complementary therapies by governments and the medical fraternity. There is evidence to suggest that an increasing number of hospital trusts are employing
therapists or allowing volunteer practitioners to provide therapies such
as massage, aromatherapy and reflexology (Graham 1998, NAHAT 1993,
Rankin-Box 1997). There is also a growing number of research projects

reporting on the use and benefits of reflexology and 'foot massage' (delivered by reflexologists and/or incorporating reflexology techniques) in hospital wards, managing pain, reducing anxiety, improving perceptions of care (Dryden et al 1998, 1999, Griffiths 1995, Hulme et al 1999). In arguing for greater use of touch therapies such as reflexology, Ashcroft (1994) has highlighed the stresses of hospitalization with acute illness; these include:

• the anxiety arising from being in an alien environment
• being disturbed constantly for clinical observations and the administration of often uncomfortable medical investigations and treatments
• fear of dislodging intravenous and monitoring equipment
• being unable to drink and eat normally
• physical discomfort made worse by wounds, immobility, invasive catheters and sleep deprivation
• intrusion from noise, light and smells
• separation from friends and family.

Reflexology, although most commonly practised in the community (Coxon 1998, Lett 2000) is now emerging as a choice for patients being cared for in mental health settings, maternity care and palliative care settings (Kohn 1999, Tiran 1996, Trousdell 1996). The chapters to follow have been written by specialist practitioners in these and other areas. It is important to recognize that these specialities have a number of factors in common, such as the inability of conventional medicine to provide effective management of difficult symptoms or the need to facilitate relaxation and reduction in anxiety. Reflexology is perhaps uniquely appropriate for patients who may not wish to undress, given that access to the feet or possibly the hands is all that is needed (Booth 1993). Reports of its use, particularly by nurses, are growing within hospital care (Rankin-Box 1997, Sahai 1993, Trevelyan 1996). Typically, these healthcare professionals have self-funded their training and are very enthusiastic about integrating reflexology within their practice settings, despite existing workloads and some reluctance to consider its value by colleagues. Despite evidence to suggest that contracts for reflexology are increasing, some healthcare trusts and individual hospitals remain reluctant to fund treatments, because of concerns about research evidence, insurance and the quality of practitioner training (Graham et al 1998). Evidence from the literature and evaluations of reflexology projects (see Chapter 5) suggest that many of these challenges can be overcome, concerns ameliorated and benefits identified for patients. The challenge to those wanting to see a more integrated or integrative service is to achieve year-by-year funding for complementary therapies. There are a number of important steps and safeguards that can assist in achieving this goal.

ESTABLISHMENT OF COMPLEMENTARY THERAPY COMMITTEES

Healthcare trusts are complex organizations with layers of administration and systems of reviewing and managing clinical practices. Reflexology, although not usually perceived as an essential provision, is none the less an intervention that requires managing and delivery by skilled practitioners. Those making referrals to practitioners, even if they are volunteers carrying out very simple treatments, are delegating treatment to patients and require to be satisfied that it is both beneficial and not harmful. At Trust Board level, members may have little or no knowledge of reflexology, by whom and how it is practised, and the extent of availability in the Trust. Surveys have been conducted on the popularity of complementary therapies and the number of contracts for services, but little quantifiable data exist on the numbers of treatments given and/or patients receiving them. An important way to share information and agree policies and protocols is the establishment of a Complementary Therapy Committee, with representation from practitioners, management and, if possible, service users. Alternatively, this work can be included in the activities of Policy and Practice Committees. These organizations can delegate to working parties such activities as audit and drafting of protocols and policies. A number of Trusts have been proactive in this work and can be approached for advice and copies of protocols and policies (Rankin-Box & McVey 2001) (see Useful addresses and contacts, p 132). Important first steps in planning any audit activities are to conduct surveys of interest in complementary therapies by patients and clinical staff, gathering information about existing complementary therapy skills and training amongst staff and preparing and revising treatment records so that data can be collected. This could include details of reasons for the referral, evaluation comments from the patient and a record of treatment times and observed responses to treatment.

INTEGRATION AND THE 'BUSYNESS' OF ACUTE HOSPITAL CARE

Hospitals have changed dramatically over the last few decades. Advances in medical practice, such as keyhole and laser surgery, have meant inpatient stays are now generally shorter. This rapid turnover, together with the complexities of treatment, has an impact on staff–patient interactions, often reducing the time available to ask questions and allay anxieties and concerns. Advances in anaesthetics have speeded physical recovery time from interventions and investigations, enabling early discharge. While this has helped to contain the rising costs of health care it can, and frequently does, mean there are greater pressures on community and family care. Being a hospitalized patient in an acute hospital can be extremely stressful and alienating. Mitzi Blennerhassett talks about her experience as a patient by likening it to being on a production line, receiving one treatment after the other, with no real communication with healthcare professionals, as if she was floating in no-man's land 'waiting for a hand to hold mine' (Blennerhassett, 1996 p 25). Reflexology can provide a means of tactile communication through which physical contact that is both therapeutic and nurturing can be made – literally holding the feet and holding the person (Fig. 9.1, Plate 11).

EVIDENCE FOR INTEGRATING REFLEXOLOGY

It has been suggested in the nursing literature that the introduction of complementary therapies, such as reflexology and foot massage in healthcare settings, could be an ideal non-pharmacological way of managing difficult symptoms, such as pain and nausea as well as reducing stress and limiting anxiety (Botting 1997, Cox & Hayes 1998, Dunn et al 1995, Grealish et al 2000, Stephenson & Weinrich 2000). Aside from the patient feeling the benefits, relatives too appear to gain satisfaction from the provision of reflexology. Dobbs (1985) describes a project to offer reflexology in an oncology unit, with patients reporting feeling less abandoned and their relatives appreciating

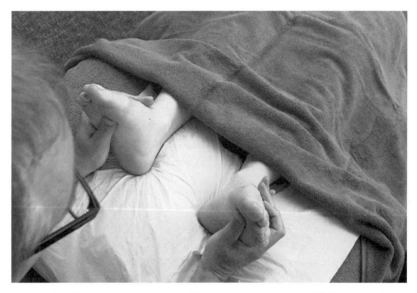

Figure 9.1 Practitioner making contact with the feet (see also Plate 11). Photo courtesy of Katie Spruce BA (Hons), medical photographer, Christie Hospital NHS Trust, with permission.

seeing something done, which helped with pain aside from medication. Cromwell et al (1999) also reported that relatives valued the provision of reflexology on a neurology unit, judging its availability to be a special treat and even sitting in on the treatments to see the benefits for themselves. Reflexology provision within a surgical unit has also been reported. Griffiths (1995) describes a reflexology project in which 52 patients on an orthopaedic ward were treated using reflexology pre- and post-hip and knee surgery. Apart from the treatments being appreciated by the patients, there was evidence that the use of postoperative analgesia was reduced. It was also reported that earlier discharges occurred in the group receiving reflexology, compared to the control conventional treatment only group.

REFLEXOLOGY IN HOSPITAL IS DIFFERENT

Patients and their relatives may appreciate the provision of reflexology in hospital but the realities of carrying out the intervention are not without challenge. It needs to be recognized that the majority of people accessing reflexology are able to travel to a clinic, pay privately and attend for a series of treatments. Although access through the public sector is growing in areas, such as maternity care hospices and cancer daycare, this often depends on the work of volunteers, limited funds, choice and availability. For healthcare practitioners using reflexology in acute admissions settings, there may be problems with continuity of the therapeutic relationship. Such everyday practical issues of competing priorities, shift patterns, staffing levels and variable length of stay for patients can dilute reflexology and other touch therapies to the status of an ad hoc 'add on' task or technique (Bay 1995). This is supported by a survey of critical care services, in which complementary therapies were not seen as routine but as provided infrequently by motivated staff (Hayes & Cox 1999). Some participants in this survey reported that consultants had actually prohibited the use of complementary therapies. This stance was seen to be due to their lack of knowledge about benefits, unsubstantiated fear of side-effects and a belief that the use of complementary and alternative therapies could undermine the medical model of care.

In orthodox settings, the potential for intruding noise levels and distractions associated with a busy clinical setting need to be taken into consideration. In measuring noise levels in one hospital department Biley (1996) reports that sluice machines can reach noise levels of 80 decibels and, when combined with other noises in a busy hospital department, was like having a 'thundering lorry' passing through (Biley 1996 p 114). In a study exploring the delivering of 61 treatments of reflexology in a ward setting, Dryden et al (1999) found interruptions, noise levels and overhead conversations alarming and distracting for the practitioners. However, for the patients these things did not appear to affect the session, it was as if their attention was focused on receiving the touch and/or it was possible that they had become tolerant of these conditions.

APPROACHES TO PROVIDING REFLEXOLOGY

Identifying when and to whom it is appropriate to offer reflexology presents challenges. Currently, provision of reflexology in acute hospital settings is largely on an ad hoc basis, delivered by existing healthcare staff or as part of a pilot or research project (Dryden et al 1999). Volunteer reflexologists may visit wards and departments, supervised by clinical staff, providing only short treatments without any remuneration to selected patients deemed suitable for treatment. Some patients also request that their own practitioners be allowed to provide private treatment whilst in hospital. It is very important that whatever arrangement is made it is done with the permission of the patient and their consultant. In most cases this will be required in writing with a record made of treatment sessions kept in the patient's hospital notes.

Finding a mutually convenient time is important, avoiding mealtimes, ward rounds and at peak visiting in the early evening. Dryden et al (1999) found that the best time to offer treatment was early afternoon, when the ward had a rest period and there were few visitors. Reflexology, like other forms of bodywork, can have a variety of benefits including assistance with physical problems, such as mobility and pain (Structural benefits), help in providing nurturing and holding (Emotional benefits) and restoring and mobilizing energy for self-healing (Energetic benefits). Mackereth (2000) has devised from these common areas the SEE model (Box 9.1) to help establish a working contract with a patient wanting a bodywork therapy. Additional practice points are overviewed in Box 9.2 and these are based on further findings from the Dryden et al (1998, 1999) project, evaluating a pilot service in a neurosciences ward. In the study, healthcare staff with training in reflexology gave treatments during their hours of work. At recorded supervision meetings, it was reported that some reflexology sessions had to be cancelled or rescheduled due to increased workload, staff sickness and more urgent priorities (Cromwell 1999).

It is understandable that some patients wanting reflexology or other therapies will look to private practitioners if ward staff are unable or are too busy. In Case study 9.1, the patient arranged for a private reflexologist to provide treatment during a hospital stay. Full or part funding is sometimes made available to patients by charitable organizations that focus on particular disease groups, such as multiple sclerosis or Parkinson's disease. This scenario demonstrates that some individuals with the financial resources can access reflexology whilst in hospital. The patient's consent and the consultant's

---

Box 9.1 The Structural, Emotional and Energetic (SEE) model for therapeutic contracts in reflexology, massage and bodywork (Mackereth 2000)

The examples given below are not exhaustive or mutually exclusive. For example, a patient might want to feel nurtured, be less anxious and sleep better.

Structural
- Reduce muscle ache and tension. e.g. after sport activity, postural problems
- Manage physical symptoms of anxiety. e.g. restlessness, insomnia
- Improve and support the cardiovascular system
- Support and maximize muscle function
- Help digestion and excretory functions
- Improve libido and sensuality
- Support for healing and prevention of illness
- Manage and improve resistance to stress.

Emotional
- Connect with feelings through/about the body
- Meet and contain potentially overwhelming emotions
- Witnessing, holding and comforting
- Nurture self-esteem and feelings of well-being
- Support process/personal development work.*

*This work would require the patient to be in psychotherapy or counselling.

Energetic*
- Acknowledge and honour depletion of energy
- Open the body to restoring and holding energy
- Release energy that is blocked
- Connect synergistically with energy in a room or between the therapist and patient using visualization/colour/ritual/symbols
- Expansion beyond and encompassing the physical body
- Pleasurable energy moving through the body 'joy unfolding'
- Strengthen energetic connection with the earth 'grounding'.

*The term 'energetic' can be interpreted to mean chi, prana or other cultural and spiritual concepts of energy.

---

agreement had been assured, but there are other issues to consider when a reflexologist makes hospital visits. First, the environment is radically different from a clinic or the patient's home; interruptions are common, with often only a curtain to separate a patient from a busy ward. In the Dryden et al (1999) study, 'do not disturb' notices and drawn curtains proved to be no barrier to staff interrupting sessions for a variety of reasons. Some patients also wanted their relatives to sit in on treatments and, although this should not be discouraged, it is necessary to ask them to sit quietly and to ask questions either before or after the session (see Case study 9.2).

MANAGEMENT AND SUPERVISORY ISSUES

Reports from the Foundation for Integrated Medicine (FIM) (1997) and the House of Lords (2000) have both made many important recommendations for the regulation and training of complementary and alternative

---

Box 9.2 Practice points for conventional healthcare settings

Preparation
- Ensure you have consent from the patient, the consultant and the ward sister/charge nurse
- Encourage the patient to inform family and/or partner that they are considering receiving reflexology
- Ensure you have made a workable contract with the patient. For example, identify how the patient might like to feel at the end of the session, e.g. relaxed or more comfortable (not a substitute for prescribed pain medication)
- Adhere to hospital infection control policies – strict hand washing, use of clean towel with each patient and correct disposal of paper towels
- Arrange a suitable time for the treatment. For example, choosing a time when neither of you will be interrupted
- Make sure that the environment and the position you are working in is comfortable at all times.

During and post-treatment
- Check intermittently that the patient is comfortable and happy to continue (ongoing consent)
- If a patient's visitor wishes to be present (and the patient agrees) make sure that the visitor is briefed beforehand to sit quietly – relatives often feel that they have to talk
- Acknowledge background noise and distractions by noticing it but coming back to the work (you can ask the patient to do likewise)
- Make sure that you can monitor the patient's post-treatment responses. For example, avoid treating a patient just before finishing your shift
- Record the treatment(s) within the patient's existing records and maintain your own confidential records.

Case study 9.1 The patient's own arrangement

Mr Grant has a neurological condition, which has now left him dependent on mechanical ventilation via a permanent tracheostomy. Arrangements are being made for home ventilation. Mr Grant has found that reflexology maintains good bowel function and helps with sleep and relaxation. He has previously paid for the treatment privately and his General Practitioner had no objections. The patient's consultant has given permission for the reflexology treatments to be continued.

Case study 9.2

Jo had numerous work colleagues, friends and family visiting her during the acute phase of her illness, a rare neurological condition that can lead to respiratory problems (Guillain–Barré syndrome). She was receiving reflexology for 30 minutes twice a week. These were often given in the afternoon when worried colleagues and family visited. They all wanted to stay with Jo and observe the treatments being given. Jo appeared to be OK with this but their constant asking of questions became disruptive and distracting. The practitioner suggested that it would be best if they asked questions before and afterwards, so that Jo could relax and have the complete attention of the therapist. This was agreed and Jo was then able to relax fully and the visitors appeared to be more comfortable just being there.

Box 9.3	Examples of reflexology provision	
Type of practitioners	**Management issues**	**Possible strategies**
Volunteer reflexologists (non-healthcare professionals)	Need to identify means of monitoring and supervising No formal contract to manage their services Variable knowledge of health and illness Provision can cease if volunteers remove their services	Employment of a complementary therapy coordinator to manage volunteers Provide in-service education and support for further training Audit service to develop a case for funded sessional work
Role expansion for healthcare staff (qualified reflexologists)	Competition with existing role and duties	Allocate set hours for the activity Different uniform and role title Consider providing reflexology in a different, but linked clinical area

medicine practitioners providing their services in healthcare settings (see Further Reading, p 132). Ideally, formal training programmes are required, with clinical placements in a variety of private and public healthcare settings, supported by supervision and assessment of competency. The history of reflexology provision has often included the valued service of dedicated volunteer reflexologists, or enthusiastic healthcare staff giving reflexology treatments as an add-on to their existing duties (Bay 1995). Box 9.3 sets out these two provisions, the managerial issues that can arise and possible strategies to best manage them. For example, Dryden et al (1999) found that nursing staff providing reflexology did not get interrupted during treatments when they wore a different uniform. At the authors's place of work, a ward sister, trained in complementary therapies, has found it necessary to wear a different uniform and provide services in another ward, so as to separate this activity from her main duties and avoid interruptions.

Coordinator/Practitioner roles for complementary therapies are beginning to emerge and these will be pivotal in managing volunteers and paid session therapists, as well as being a resource for healthcare staff and patients. The role can also include facilitating and organizing in-service training courses and income-generating through consultative and education work. Another important aspect of this role (and of the Complementary Therapy Committee, where one is in place) is the auditing of existing or piloted services. This activity, along with evidence from literature reviews, can help to build proposals for securing permanent funding for complementary and alternative medicine therapies, such as reflexology.

CONCLUSION

This chapter is an introduction to the second section of this book. It has identified key issues with regard to providing, evaluating and managing reflexology services in hospital departments and daycare services. It is likely that, in the future, many more specialist clinical areas will see an expansion in reflexology provision. Research projects that report benefits for patients (see also Chapter 5) have been identified and suggest best practice when planning and delivering treatments in clinical settings.

The following recommendations have been made in order to support the development of clinical reflexology; Chapters 10–14 will explore specific issues related to specialist care and reflexology:

RECOMMENDATIONS FOR DEVELOPING AND INTEGRATING REFLEXOLOGY IN CLINICAL PRACTICE

- Evaluate hospital provision of reflexology for benefits and find the best ways of delivering treatment through quality research and audit activities.
- Presentation of conference papers, workshops and poster sessions on complementary therapies, such as reflexology, covering various specialities.
- Share best practice in reflexology in journals covering a wide range of clinical areas, e.g. intensive care, accident and emergency, and orthopaedics.
- Establish and/or participate in complementary therapy/reflexology networks and specialist interest groups to obtain support and share best practice.
- Establish and/or participate in a Trust or hospital's Complementary Therapy Committee.
- Ensure that only qualified complementary therapists with experience in managing patient care in the private and public healthcare sectors are employed.
- Support practitioners to complete courses in specialist application.
- Provide and support supervision and management arrangements for all practitioners providing reflexology, for example, by employment of a Complementary Therapy Coordinator/Practitioner.

REFERENCES

Ashcroft R. Complementary therapy in the critical care unit. In: Millar B, Burnard P, eds. Critical care nursing: caring for the critically ill adult. London: Baillière Tindall; 1994.

Bay F. Complementary therapies – just another task? Complementary Therapies in Nursing and Midwifery 1995; 1(1):34–36.

Biley F. Hospitals: healing environments? Complementary Therapies in Nursing and Midwifery 1996; 2(2):110–115.

Blennerhassett M. The pain of the gentle touch. Health Service Journal 1996; 11 April:25.

Booth B. Complementary therapies. London: Nursing Times/MacMillan Press; 1993.

Botting D. Review of the literature on the effectiveness of reflexology. Complementary Therapies in Nursing and Midwifery 1997; 3(5):125–130.

Cox C, Hayes J. Experiences of administrating and receiving therapeutic touch in intensive care. Complementary Therapies in Nursing and Midwifery 1998; 3:163–167.

Coxon T. Reflexology in the community. International Journal of Alternative and Complementary Medicine 1998; May:14–16.

Cromwell C, Dryden S, Jones D, Mackereth P. 'Just the ticket'; case studies, reflections and clinical supervision (Part III). Complementary Therapies in Nursing and Midwifery 1999; 5(2):42–45.

Dobbs BZ. Alternative health approaches. Nursing Mirror 1985; 160(9):41–42.

Dryden S, Holden S, Mackereth P. 'Just the ticket'; integrating massage and reflexology in practice (Part I). Complementary Therapies in Nursing and Midwifery 1998; 4(6):154–159.

Dryden S, Holden S, Mackereth P. 'Just the ticket'; the findings of a pilot complementary therapy service (Part II). Complementary Therapies in Nursing and Midwifery 1999; 5(1):15–18.

Dunn C, Sleep J, Collett D. Sensing an improvement: an experimental study to evaluate the use of aromatherapy, massage and periods of rest in an intensive care unit. Journal of Advanced Nursing 1995; 21(1):34–40.

Foundation for Integrated Medicine (FIM). Integrated healthcare – a way forward for the next five years? London: FIM; 1997.

Graham L, Goldstone L, Ejindu A et al. Penetration of complementary therapies into NHS trust and private hospital practice. Complementary Therapies in Nursing and Midwifery 1998; 4(6):160–165.

Grealish L, Lomasney A, Whiteman B. Foot massage: a nursing intervention to modify the distressing symptoms of pain and nausea in patients hospitalised with cancer. Cancer Nursing 2000; 23(3):237–243.

Griffiths P. Reflexology. In: Rankin-Box D, ed. The nurses's handbook of complementary therapies. London: Churchill Livingstone; 1995.

Hayes JA, Cox CL. The integration of complementary therapies in North and South Thames Regional Health Authorities' critical care units. Complementary Therapies in Nursing and Midwifery 1999; 5(4):103–107.

House of Lords. Select Committee on Science and Technology. Complementary and alternative medicine (HL Paper 123). London: HMSO; 2000.

Hulme J, Waterman H, Hillier VF. The effects of foot massage on patients' perception of care following laparoscopic sterilization as day case patients. Journal of Advanced Nursing 1999; 30(2):460–468.

Kohn M. Complementary therapies. London: Macmillan Cancer Relief; 1999.

Lett A. Reflex zone therapy for health professionals. London: Churchill Livingstone; 2000.

National Association of Health Authorities and Trusts (NAHAT). Complementary therapies in the NHS (Research Paper. No. 10). London: NAHAT; 1993.

Rankin-Box D. Therapies in practice: a survey assessing nurses' use of complementary therapies. Complementary Therapies in Nursing and Midwifery 1997; 3(4):92–99.

Rankin B, McVey M. Policy development. In: Rankin-Box D, ed. The nurse's handbook of complementary therapies. 2nd edn. London: Harcourt Publishers; 2001.

Sahai CM. Reflexology – its place in modern healthcare. Professional Nurse 1993; 8(11):722–725.

Stephenson NLN, Weinrich SP. The effects of foot reflexology on anxiety and pain in patients with breast and lung cancer. Oncology Nursing Forum 2000; 27(1):67–72.

Stone J. How might traditional remedies be incorporated into discussions of integrated medicine? Complementary Therapies in Nursing and Midwifery 2000; 7(2):55–58.

Tiran D. The use of complementary therapies in midwifery practice: a focus on reflexology. Complementary Therapies in Nursing and Midwifery 1996; 2:32–37.

Trevelyan J. A true complement. Nursing Times 1996; 92:5.
Trousdell P. Reflexology meets emotional needs. International Journal of Alternative and Complementary Medicine 1996; November: 9–12.

FURTHER READING

NHS Confederation. Complementary medicine in the NHS: managing the issues (Research paper No. 4). London: NHS Confederation; 1997.

USEFUL ADDRESSES

Peter Mackereth
Chair, Complementary Therapy Committee, Christie Hospital, Wilmslow Road, Withington, Manchester, M20 4BX
Tel: 0161 446 3795

10

Supporting women during pregnancy and childbirth

Denise Tiran

Abstract

This chapter explores the uses, safety, precautions and potential complications of using reflexology during pregnancy and childbirth. The legal implications for practitioners who are not qualified midwives are discussed, placing emphasis firmly on professional accountability.

Key words: safety, accountability, integration

There has been much controversy about whether reflexology should be administered to pregnant women, particularly during the first trimester (Hall 1991, Marquardt 2000). There is no research evidence to support this practice and reflexologists are understandably cautious when treating women who are pregnant, with some declining to treat them at all. Reasons given for this caution include the perceived risk of affecting fetal development (Crane 1997) or inducing spontaneous abortion, preterm labour or antepartum haemorrhage. There is no evidence or theoretical basis for the misguided belief that malformations of the embryo could occur during the first trimester. Similarly, although reflexology can indeed be used to stimulate uterine contractions at term (see p 143), it must be stressed that therapeutically appropriate reflexology will *not* cause pregnancy complications.

However, reflexology is a powerful tool that, when used accurately, can have positive effects. By inference, therefore, if it is used without due regard for safety it could lead to undesired reactions. Loss of a pregnancy in the first trimester occurs naturally as a result of physiopathological or psychological factors and there is no research evidence available to confirm or deny that reflexology could cause abortion. However, women who suffer miscarriage often strive to find a reason for it and may, in the absence of any other aetiology, attribute the cause to reflexology. It is therefore wise to act with caution, especially during the first trimester and particularly if the therapist is not also a midwife or doctor. It is also necessary to acknowledge that any reflexology performed during pregnancy must take account of the fact that both the client *and* her fetus are being treated.

REFLEXOLOGY DURING PREGNANCY

Reflexologists who are not also qualified midwives, obstetricians or general practitioners *must* recognize the limitations of their own professional accountability. It is illegal for anyone other than a midwife or doctor, or one in training under supervision, to take sole responsibility for the care of expectant and labouring women except in an emergency. Thus any reflexology given at this time must be complementary rather than alternative to conventional maternity care and, in the view of this author, is best integrated into the conventional maternity services by being provided by the midwives who are already caring for the woman. As with other complementary therapies, practitioners of reflexology may feel that caring for this client group is pleasant, productive and often very lucrative. However, those in independent practice who wish to specialize in providing care for pregnant women must ensure that they have a thorough understanding of pregnancy physiology, embryonic and fetal development, potential maternal and fetal pathology and the current maternity services (see Case study 10.1). At the very least this should include a knowledge of the first aid treatment that may be necessary if a woman has a precipitate labour, antepartum haemorrhage, eclamptic fit or cord prolapse following spontaneous rupture of the membranes.

Unfortunately, even some of the reflexology texts written by well-known experts fail to demonstrate adequate understanding to equip themselves or their readers to treat pregnant women safely and, indeed, some are dangerously inaccurate. Readers are referred to the list of Further Reading (page 145) for suitable texts on maternity care. (*Note*: only *midwives* can provide *midwifery* care [the title 'midwife' is protected in statute]; all other professionals offer *maternity* care.)

PRECAUTIONS

Pregnancy is a normal physiological condition for the majority of expectant mothers and receiving reflexology at this time is safe when undertaken by

---

Case study 10.1 Laura

Laura was receiving regular reflexology from the complementary therapy (CT) midwife to keep her blood pressure within normal limits, as it had been very high in her previous pregnancy. At her 32-week appointment she arrived looking generally unwell, stating that her ankles had been very swollen 4 days before and that she had had a headache, but had done nothing about it. Her headache persisted and her ankles remained very oedematous. On questioning, Laura said she felt sick, had visual disturbance and right-sided epigastric pain, all symptoms of fulminating pre-eclampsia. The CT midwife took her blood pressure, which was pathologically high, and then went to confer with a colleague regarding relevant blood tests to exclude further complications. On her return Laura said she felt a sudden pounding behind her eyes, and her skin had turned grey. The midwife became alarmed, assessing Laura as possibly about to have an eclamptic fit, and rushed to transfer her to the delivery suite. On investigation, it transpired that Laura had a severe urinary tract infection that was mimicking impending eclampsia. This was treated immediately by the medical staff to prevent preterm labour commencing.

The point at issue here is not that the midwife was mistaken in her diagnosis but that, taking into account the speed with which Laura's condition deteriorated, the midwife was alert enough to act swiftly on the assumption of one of the most serious complications of pregnancy. This demonstrates the need to understand fully the pathophysiology of pregnancy and to work in conjunction with the conventional maternity services.

---

a qualified therapist experienced in treating the particular client group. There are very few contraindications additional to those relevant to all clients, although extra care should be taken when treating women with complications of pregnancy that require medical care (Box 10.1). Reflexologists who are in any doubt regarding the appropriateness of treating a particular client should refrain from doing so unless and until they have sought the relevant advice.

One of the possible problems associated with the increasing popularity of complementary therapies is that one or more therapies may be used in combination. Where an individual practitioner's method of working incorporates other therapies, such as acupressure or aromatherapy alongside reflexology, it is *vital* that the therapist understands fully the application of the additional therapies to pregnant and childbearing women. For example,

---

Box 10.1 Pregnancy conditions in which reflexology should be used with extreme caution or avoided

- History of repeated spontaneous abortions
- Preterm labour or spontaneous membrane rupture in this or a previous pregnancy
- Previous stillbirth or history of intrauterine growth retardation in this or a previous pregnancy
- Antepartum haemorrhage in this or a previous pregnancy
- Pre-eclampsia, eclampsia or severe pre-existing essential hypertension
- Multiple pregnancy
- Breech presentation, transverse or unstable lie
- Medical conditions exacerbated by pregnancy, e.g. cardiac disease, diabetes

Crane (1997) advocates the incorporation of acupressure techniques, some of which are incorrectly identified as safe to use in pregnancy. This author has had communication with midwives who had been taught additional techniques but who failed to appreciate that they were, in fact, stimulating acupressure points. Some reflexologists may administer essential oils as part of their treatment, but many of these are contraindicated during pregnancy and childbirth (Tiran 2000). All practitioners, both conventional and complementary, should be able to justify their actions, supported by research-based evidence where available, and it is inappropriate and potentially professionally suicidal, especially in this age of litigation, to act without full knowledge, understanding and experience of the therapies and the client group.

THE BENEFITS OF REFLEXOLOGY IN PREGNANCY AND CHILDBIRTH

Women who actively choose to receive regular reflexology during pregnancy have been shown to gain a degree of relaxation that indirectly impacts on the developing fetus (Motha & McGrath 1993). Some women may have been attending for treatment prior to conception and may even have sought help for infertility, subfertility or premenstrual syndrome. Anovulatory infertility may be resolved through the stimulation of the reflex zones for the pituitary gland and ovaries (see Fig. 10.1), whilst general relaxing reflexology can be helpful where stress and anxiety appear to be contributory factors. Oleson & Flocco (1993) showed significant responses to premenstrual symptoms in women who received foot, hand and ear reflexology, which may indicate its value in times of hormonal upheaval. Simply receiving regular manual therapy from a practitioner whom they come to know can be very beneficial for some women, providing an opportunity to discuss their worries and concerns, but again, therapists should not offer any advice or treatment for which they are not adequately trained.

Stress, tension, anxiety and fear affect every pregnant woman to a greater or lesser degree. Reflexology can have profound benefits at this time, although whether this is due to the physical effects of reflexology, the therapeutic value of human touch or the psychological effects of interaction with the therapist is debatable. It is, however, this latter aspect that makes it so vital that the therapist has a sound knowledge-base regarding pregnancy and childbirth, as eye-to-eye contact facilitates discussion and enables the mother to ask questions and raise concerns, especially when treatment is offered on a regular basis so that the expectant mother comes to know her therapist well. This author frequently finds that women receiving regular reflex zone therapy raise a range of personal and intimate concerns, such as sexual and relationship difficulties during pregnancy. It would not, however,

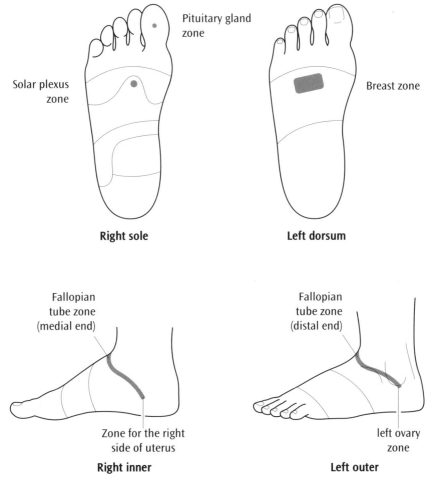

Figure 10.1   Reflexology map showing some areas of relevance to conception, pregnancy and lactation.

be within the realm of responsibility of a reflexologist who is not also a midwife, nurse or health visitor to attempt to advise the woman on these subjects.

POSITIONING FOR REFLEXOLOGY DURING PREGNANCY AND CHILDBIRTH

It is preferable to position the woman sitting up or in a semi-recumbent position to enable her to converse if she wishes, but also to prevent the effects of supine hypotension from lying flatter, especially in later pregnancy. Care should be taken at the end of the treatment to ensure that the woman does not experience further hypotension from sitting or standing up too quickly. Many women feel slightly dizzy or faint, particularly after the first treatment, and some will become nauseous while the treatment is ongoing. It is better to discontinue the current treatment if this occurs, to avoid additional reactions.

If the woman has chosen to lie flatter, it is important, at the end of the treatment, to assist her in rising from the couch by advising her to turn onto her side and then push herself up to a sitting position, wait a few seconds and then stand. This avoids the danger of overstretching the pelvic ligaments or causing pain in the sacroiliac joint area, both of which are influenced by the hormones progesterone and relaxin during pregnancy. It will also prevent postural hypotension, which is more common at this time.

During labour, it may be necessary to perform reflex zone therapy with the woman in whatever position she has adopted for most comfort, for example, lying on her side, kneeling on all fours or standing upright. It is unlikely that a full treatment will be given during labour and the therapist must adapt in accordance with the woman's preferences, sometimes even refraining from undertaking the treatment. Similarly, during the early postnatal period the woman may be in bed or sitting in a chair and treatment will need to be planned accordingly.

REFLEXOLOGY DURING THE ANTENATAL PERIOD

Specific physiological disorders of pregnancy can be treated effectively with reflexology or reflex zone therapy (Box 10.2). It is not always essential to undertake a complete reflexology treatment; indeed, the nature of the clinical NHS work of this author is such that short, focused manipulations of the relevant reflex zones have been found to be equally as effective in relieving symptoms as full treatments, which contradicts normal practice (see also Chapter 5). Some physiological conditions respond with just one

---

Box 10.2 Physiological conditions of pregnancy that may respond to reflexology

- Nausea and vomiting
- Headache and migraine
- Backache, sciatica, sacroiliac joint pain
- Symphysis pubis diastasis
- Constipation and diarrhoea
- Haemorrhoids
- Varicose veins
- Heartburn and indigestion
- Ptyalism (excessive salivation)
- Carpal tunnel syndrome
- Retention of urine from retroverted incarcerated gravid uterus
- Stress, anxiety, muscle tension

or two treatments of no more than 10 minutes duration, with no further appointments being necessary. These include nausea and vomiting, constipation, carpal tunnel syndrome and heartburn. This does imply that the method of reflexology is used in more of a reductionist manner, simply offering additional strategies for dealing with specific problems, but demonstrates its value in integrated maternity care.

NAUSEA AND VOMITING

It is the experience of this author that women who suffer severe nausea and vomiting in pregnancy frequently have a history of neck or back problems, such as a previous whiplash injury to the cervical vertebrae or ongoing lumbosacral discomfort, probably as a result of minor vertebral displacement. Although these may cause no real pain when the woman is not pregnant, the relaxation of the joints and ligaments caused by the pregnancy hormones relaxin and progesterone often exacerbates the conditions. Reflex zone therapy to the foot areas for the head, neck and spine can be especially valuable in relieving the intensity of nausea and frequency of vomiting. Incorporation of treatment to the zones for the shoulders will reduce any tension of the muscles, which can occur as a result of constantly leaning forwards to vomit. Treatment may also be effective because of working the foot zones incorporating the vagus nerve area of the neck and the brain zone, including the vomiting centre. Crane (1997) suggests that it is the working of the oesophagus zone to combat heartburn, indigestion and acid reflux that assists in relieving the sickness, but this shows a singular lack of understanding of the variable gestations at which these two symptoms occur.

In some women the condition is so debilitating that other complementary treatments may be necessary, such as P6 acupuncture/acupressure (Belluomini et al 1994; de Aloysio & Penacchioni 1992), specific safe essential oils (Tiran 2000) or herbal remedies (Stapleton & Tiran 2000), homeopathy (Cummings 2000), osteopathy (Conway 2000) or chiropractic (Tellefsen 2000). A few women require hospital admission with hyperemesis gravidarum for the relevant pharmacological treatment, although reflexology can be used as a relaxing adjunct to conventional management (Case study 10.2).

HEADACHE AND MIGRAINE

Many women experience headaches in early pregnancy caused by the vasodilatation of the cerebral blood vessels by progesterone. Regular reflexology may alleviate both the intensity and the duration of the headaches and has been found, in some client groups, to be at least as effective as analgesia but without the accompanying side-effects (Lafuente et al

---

Case study 10.2 Gina

Gina had suffered severe hyperemesis in both her previous pregnancies but this time the problem was worse. She vomited up to 10 times daily and had already been admitted to hospital for rehydration seven times by the 16th week of pregnancy. She attended the complementary therapy (CT) midwife clinic, accompanied by her mother, who walked with a stick. Gina had had a history of neck and back pain before pregnancy and was complaining of lower abdominal pain, for which no cause could be found. On examining her feet, the CT midwife immediately noticed a brown pigmented area over the lower aspect of the inner ankle bone on Gina's left foot, an area corresponding to the symphysis pubis. On closer questioning, it transpired that Gina's 'abdominal' pain was in fact suprapubic and, from a midwifery perspective, seemed to be in keeping with symphysis pubis diastasis. Gina also said that she felt tenderness when the midwife palpated the lower edge of the outer ankle bone on the same foot, the area relating to the hip and sacroiliac joint. The CT midwife intuitively asked Gina's mother the reason for her use of a stick and was told that she had been born with no acetabulum, a fact that was only discovered at the age of 31 when a pelvic X-ray was performed. The CT midwife returned to Gina's feet, working on the spine, neck, hip, sacroiliac joint and symphysis pubis zones. Gina could tolerate only a few minutes' work but reported feeling much better, less nauseated and relieved of much of the pain in her lower abdomen.

The following week Gina arrived looking dreadful and said she had been so severely sick that she had been readmitted to hospital 5 days after the reflexology. However, she agreed to further treatment and again left the clinic feeling much more at ease, both physically and psychologically. On the third week Gina required virtually no reflexology – the vomiting had decreased to just a couple of times a day and the perpetual nausea had ceased. Gina was delighted, needed no further treatment and progressed with her pregnancy with no other complications.

Following delivery, Gina underwent investigations and was found to have an acetabular problem similar to that of her mother, for which she was then able to have treatment.

1990; Launso et al 1999). The frequency of treatments is worthy of consideration: this author has a heavily oversubscribed weekly clinic held on a Monday and many women seem to obtain relief from their headaches until Friday of each week, that is, for 5 days after treatment. It is not clear whether this indicates the need for treatment to be repeated every 5 days or whether the change of activity for most people over weekends triggers further headaches.

Treatment of women complaining of headaches, particularly in later pregnancy, must always be accompanied by a midwifery or medical examination to exclude fulminating pre-eclampsia or impending eclampsia, although it is also possible that hypertensive disorders of pregnancy may respond to reflexology treatment (Yongsheng & Xiaolian 1995).

BACKACHE AND SCIATICA

Similar findings regarding frequency of treatments arise when treating women suffering lumbosacral backache, with associated sacroiliac pain and sciatica. The discomfort usually intensifies as the weight and lumbar lordosis increase throughout pregnancy; the earlier reflexology is required for backache the more likely it is that treatment will not be fully effective and women may best be referred to an osteopath or chiropractor. It is noticeable that foot zones for the sacroiliac joints are usually tender in most pregnant women, probably due to the ongoing hormonal effects. Although some minor symptomatic relief can be obtained with reflexology in women with symphysis pubis diastasis, this is most effectively treated with chiropractic (Tellefsen 2000).

CONSTIPATION

Constipation is a common physiological phenomenon in pregnancy and responds extremely well to reflex zone therapy (Case study 10.3), especially when combined with foot massage using a 1% blend of essential oils, such as the citrus essences or marjoram, although purists may find the mixing of therapies a contentious issue and reflexologists who are not also aromatherapists should seek help to ensure correct administration of the oils (Tiran 2000). Expectant mothers and their partners can easily be shown how to perform clockwise massage of the arches of the feet, corresponding to the large and small intestine zones. This is also an effective treatment that mothers can administer for neonatal constipation or colic. Certainly, constipation in non-pregnant patients has been shown to respond well to reflexology (Eriksen 1992). A simple home remedy that women could try is to roll the feet over two bottles resting in the arches of the feet, which provides a form of massage to the foot zones for the intestines.

CARPAL TUNNEL SYNDROME

Tingling and pain in the fingers combined with an inability to grip or perform pincer movements is due to oedema around the nerve channel in the wrists and can occur in late pregnancy, particularly at night. Reflexology can offer some temporary relief in most cases (Case study 10.4) and may be effective enough to prevent a return to the symptoms, by stimulating lymphatic and circulatory flow. Additionally, relief may be obtained by releasing

---

Case study 10.3   Rebecca

Rebecca came to see the CT midwife at 22 weeks of pregnancy complaining of constipation and said she had not had her bowels open for 3 weeks. Not surprisingly, she felt dreadful, almost toxic. The midwife performed 10 minutes of reflex zone therapy on two occasions and Rebecca reported bowel movements twice weekly. The treatment was continued regularly to maintain peristaltic action and keep Rebecca comfortable throughout the remainder of the pregnancy, sometimes combined with essential oils or homeopathic remedies when reflexology alone was not sufficient.

Case Study 10.4   Ali

Ali was a clinically obese girl who reported to the CT midwife at 28 weeks with incapacitating carpal tunnel syndrome, which severely compromised her daily life. Hers was one of the worst cases of carpal tunnel syndrome seen by the midwife who needed to see Ali weekly for the duration of her pregnancy just to keep the discomfort within manageable limits. Treatment was combined with essential oils, homeopathy and acupressure and Ali was taught how to perform reflex zone 'first aid' when the problem kept her awake at night. An added advantage of seeing her so regularly was that discussion of various concurrent psychosocial problems could take place and other physiological complaints could be treated early. Ali's carpal tunnel syndrome was so severe that she required surgery after delivery to correct it more permanently.

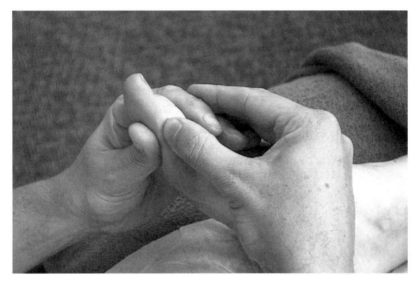

Figure 10.2   Practitioner working the neck area (see also Plate 12). Photo courtesy of Katie Spruce BA (Hons), medical photographer, Christie Hospital NHS Trust, with permission.

tensions in the neck by working on the big toes, especially if there is any suspicion of nerve involvement (Fig. 10.2, Plate 12).

INDUCTION OF LABOUR

Starting labour artificially should only be undertaken for specific reasons. It is not the role of either an independent reflexologist or a midwife/reflexologist to induce labour: it is a medical procedure that carries certain risks and is outside the scope of midwifery practice unless consultant permission has been granted. Many women request independent therapists of complementary medicine to induce labour merely because they are past their due dates, without either the woman or the therapist understanding the reasons why labour has not yet commenced or the potential complications of attempting to start labour artificially. This author believes it is *professionally irresponsible* for independent therapists to agree to stimulate uterine contractions unless adequate consultation has taken place between the therapist, the woman and the midwife or obstetrician.

However, theoretically, it is possible to initiate contractions using reflex zone therapy and this author, a practising midwife, has had agreement from consultant obstetricians in the local maternity unit to perform reflexology on specifically identified women in order to encourage the onset of labour.

Prediction of the imminence of labour is also possible with reflex zone therapy. Over many years of examining the feet of pregnant women, this author has developed the skill of estimating whether or not labour is imminent by palpating the foot zones for the anterior and posterior pituitary gland and applying the findings to a knowledge of hormonal changes in late pregnancy. Whether or not some intuitive midwifery assessment adds to the accuracy of the prediction is difficult to state, but the situation is worthy of formal investigation.

REFLEXOLOGY DURING LABOUR

Reflexology can be extremely relaxing, pain relieving and psychologically comforting during labour, although it is also necessary to bear in mind that some women dislike being touched in labour and will therefore not wish to receive reflexology at this time.

Reflexology during labour may be provided by the midwife caring for the woman as an adjunct to normal care, or the woman may have requested the presence of a reflexologist at the birth. If she is having her baby at home, this is fairly easily arranged, but if the baby is to be born in hospital the therapist will need to make the necessary arrangements early in pregnancy. This includes obtaining permission from the midwife or consultant obstetrician to be present on hospital premises. Personal professional indemnity insurance cover is essential and independent practitioners may be required to sign a form to confirm that they will not attempt to use the hospital's vicarious liability insurance in the event of a claim for negligence being brought against them. A reflexologist who is not the designated midwife must acknowledge that the midwife retains responsibility, in law, for the overall care of the mother and baby and, if necessary, the therapist may need to discontinue treatment if complications occur.

Reflexology in labour can be given for overall relaxation and stress relief, in which case a general treatment will be administered. Specific areas can be treated for pain relief; simple pressure applied to the heels can be very effective during contractions. Midwives in Denmark regularly use reflexology whilst caring for labouring women and Feder et al (1993) have shown that it can reduce the length of the first stage. Stimulation of the pituitary gland zones can accelerate the frequency and increase the strength of contractions where labour is slow, but this should only be performed by reflexologists who are fully familiar with labour physiology and the precise details of the mother's progress. Other techniques can be administered to alleviate nausea and vomiting and stress, anxiety and panic.

It is unlikely that treatment will be continued during the second stage of labour, but reflexology can be helpful in the third stage. However, it is not appropriate for an independent therapist to interfere with the progress of placental separation and delivery, whether this is passively or actively managed by the midwife, unless invited to do so. Reflex zone therapy can stimulate the separation of a normally adherent, but retained, placenta but will not be effective if the placenta is morbidly adherent, and indeed could trigger postpartum haemorrhage. However, haemorrhage could be managed in part with reflexology as an additional treatment to the usual oxytocic drugs.

POSTNATAL REFLEXOLOGY

Following delivery, reflexology can be used to treat women with physiological disorders of the puerperium, including constipation, haemorrhoids, perineal discomfort and inadequate lactation (see Chapter 11). Relief from ongoing discomfort following epidural anaesthesia, such as backache, neck pain or headache, can also be obtained (Tiran 1996).

Babies and infants respond well to reflexology or other touch therapies and minor problems such as colic and wind can be treated. The use of reflexology for neonates in intensive care is explored in Chapter 11.

CONCLUSION

Reflexology offers a gentle yet powerful tool for assisting women during pregnancy, labour and the postnatal period. It can be performed regularly for general health and wellbeing, or intermittently for specific disorders and discomforts, as well as for relief of pain, anxiety and other symptoms during labour. Practitioners who specialize in using reflexology to treat pregnant and childbearing women *must* have a thorough knowledge and understanding of physiological changes and possible complications, as well as an appreciation of the conventional maternity services. Reflexology for this client group is complementary to any orthodox maternity care provided.

REFERENCES

Belluomini J, Litt RC, Lee KA et al. Acupressure for nausea and vomiting of pregnancy: a randomized blinded study. Obstetrics and Gynaecology 1994; 84(2):245–248.
Conway P. Osteopathy during pregnancy. In Tiran D, Mack S, eds. Complementary therapies for pregnancy and childbirth. 2nd edn. London: Baillière Tindall; 2000: 39–60.
Crane B. Reflexology: the definitive practitioner's manual. Shaftesbury, Dorset: Element Books; 1997.
Cummings B. Homeopathy for pregnancy and childbirth. In Tiran D, Mack S, eds. Complementary therapies for pregnancy and childbirth. 2nd edn. London: Baillière Tindall; 2000: 13–38.
De Aloysio D, Penacchioni P. Morning sickness control in early pregnancy by Neiguan point acupressure. Obstetrics and Gynaecology 1992; 80(5):852–854.
Eriksen L. Zoneterapi mod kronisk forstoppelse (Zone therapy for chronic constipation). Sygeplejersken 1992; 92(26):7.
Feder E, Liisberg GB, Lenstrup C et al. Zone therapy in relation to birth. Proceedings of the International Confederation of Midwives 23rd International Congress 1993; 2:651–656.
Hall NM. Reflexology: a way to better health. Bath: Gateway Books; 1991.
Lafuente A, Noguera M, Puy C et al. Reflexonenbehandlung am Fuss bezuglich der prophylaktischen Behandlung bei Cephalea-Kopfschmerzen leidenen. Erfahrungsheilkunde 1990; 39:713–715.
Launso L, Brendstrup E, Amberg S. An exploratory study of reflexological treatment for headache. Alternative Therapies in Health and Medicine 1999; 5(3):57–65.
Marquardt H. Reflexotherapy of the feet. Stuttgart: Thieme; 2000. (Translation into English of the 4th German edition of 1999.)
Motha G, McGrath J. The effects of reflexology on labour outcomes. Reflexions. Journal of Association of Reflexologists 1993; 2–4.
Oleson T, Flocco W. Randomized controlled study of premenstrual symptoms treated with ear, hand and foot reflexology. Obstetrics and Gynaecology 1993; 82(6):906–911.
Stapleton H, Tiran D. Herbal medicine. In: Tiran D, Mack S, eds. Complementary therapies for pregnancy and childbirth. 2nd edn. London: Baillière Tindall; 2000:105–128.
Tellefsen T. The chiropractic approach to health care during pregnancy. In: Tiran D, Mack S, eds. Complementary therapies for pregnancy and childbirth. 2nd edn. London: Baillière Tindall; 2000: 61–78.
Tiran D. The use of complementary therapies in midwifery practice: a focus on reflexology. Complementary Therapies in Nursing and Midwifery 1996; 2:32–37.
Tiran D. Clinical aromatherapy for pregnancy and childbirth. 2nd edn. London: Harcourt Health Sciences; 2000.
Yongsheng Xu, Xiaolian S. Hypertension of pregnancy treated with foot reflexology – a case report. China Reflexology Symposium Report. Ankang City, Shaanxi: Foot Reflexology Service Centre; 1995:68.

FURTHER READING

Sweet B, Tiran D (Eds.) Mayes' Midwifery. 12th edn. London: Baillière Tindall; 1997. This textbook for midwives gives in-depth research-based information about pregnancy physiology, management and services.
Tiran D. Natural remedies for morning sickness and other pregnancy problems. London: Quadrille Publishing; 2001. Provides an overview of a range of complementary therapies of use during pregnancy and childbirth, with accompanying explanations of physiology, aimed at expectant mothers.

USEFUL ADDRESSES

Complementary Maternity Forum
c/o Denise Tiran, Principal Lecturer – Complementary Medicine, School of Health, The
University of Greenwich, Avery Hill University Campus, Mansion Site, Bexley Road, Eltham,
London, SE9 2UG.
Tel: 0208 331 8494
Fax: 0208 331 9926
E-mail: M.D.Tiran@gre.ac.uk

11

Practising in the neonatal area

Liz Tipping

Touch and reflexology in the neonate	**Conclusion**
Stress factors in the neonatal unit	**References**
Breastfeeding in the neonatal unit	**Further reading**

Abstract

This chapter considers the value of practising reflexology specifically for parents of babies in the neonatal special and intensive care unit. The fragile nature of babies admitted to the neonatal special or intensive care unit means that it is not appropriate to consider the use of reflexology until they are well enough to be discharged, particularly as they will require highly technical medical treatments. Even then, reflexology interventions would need to be adapted and evaluated carefully as to their benefits and risks. In the absence of evidence as to the safety, let alone the efficacy of reflexology, it is highly unlikely that parents would consent to their babies receiving treatment at this time, and medical staff would rightly add justifiable concerns regarding interactions with physiological changes or drugs to any scepticism they might already have about reflexology. However, the therapy can offer a valuable adjunct to the care of the parents of babies in the neonatal unit, especially the mothers, and this chapter focuses on using reflexology for the management of maternal stress and the facilitation of lactation.

Key words: touch, stress and coping, lactation

Care in the neonatal special and intensive care unit involves not only the physiopathological care of the baby but also the emotional and psychological care of the parents, siblings and other family members. Early postnatal physical care of the mother is undertaken by the midwives on the postnatal wards or in the mother's own home if she has been discharged; it is not carried out in the neonatal unit except in an emergency. However, those physiopathological factors that affect the care of the baby, such as the initiation of breastfeeding or the ability of the mother to nurse her baby comfortably after a possibly traumatic delivery, will be of concern to the neonatal nurses and midwives who choose to work in the unit. The use of reflexology for the care of mothers during a normal postnatal recovery is dealt with in Chapter 10.

TOUCH AND REFLEXOLOGY IN THE NEONATE

Reflexology provides a valuable form of touch for more mature and healthy babies and much has been written regarding the use of positive touch, in the form of massage, for preterm and sick infants. For example, there is evidence of improvement in the infant–parent relationship when babies in the neonatal intensive care unit have received regular massage (Walker 1995; White-Traut & Nelson 1988) as this helps the parents to become more confident at handling their tiny sick baby. Tiffany Field in Miami has been instrumental in increasing the awareness of professionals and parents of the value of infant massage and has developed a system of TAC-TIC therapy (Touching and Caressing, Tender in Caring) (Adamson-Macedo et al 1993, 1994a, b, De Roiste & Bushnell 1995, De Roiste et al 1995). Touch has been found to enhance growth and maturation in the preterm infant (Field et al 1986, Kuhn et al 1991) and to stimulate greater intellectual development in children born prematurely (Adamson-Macedo et al 1993). Contrary to hitherto strongly held professional views that touching preterm babies adversely affects oxygen saturation levels, this does not seem to be the case (Adamson-Macedo et al 1997) and this research has challenged the previous policy of 'minimal handling' of these babies. Touch also appears to facilitate temperature maintenance in ill babies (Johanson et al 1992) and to have positive effects on heart rate and respiratory functioning (Harrison et al 1990, Helders et al 1988) and on sympathetic and adrenocortical functions (Acolet et al 1993, Kuhn et al 1991).

Lett (2000) suggests that reflexology can be given to healthy full-term infants on the feet, hands or back but cites contraindications such as hyperpyrexia, venous or lymphatic inflammation, localized infection at the preferred reflexology site or distress during the procedure. Lett (2000) implies that reflexology/reflex zone therapy is permissible for preterm and ill neonates and, theoretically, this author would concur with this. However, it is essential to acknowledge the power of the therapy, perhaps as yet not fully recognized, and performing reflexology on these infants requires a thorough understanding of the physiological and pathological processes of each individual baby's condition.

The simple fact that babies in the neonatal special and intensive care unit are receiving highly technical and precise medical treatment indicates that it is inappropriate to attempt reflexology therapy without permission from the paediatric consultant (as well as the parents). The practitioner must understand exactly how each of the reflexology techniques used could affect the baby's physiology and apply this knowledge to an in-depth appreciation of the baby's current condition. For example, many preterm babies remain severely jaundiced for some time as a result of the immature liver's inability to conjugate bilirubin. An inexperienced reflexologist could be tempted to stimulate the liver reflex zone in the belief that this would increase production of the enzyme gluceronyl transferase, and therefore the excretion of fetal haemoglobin, without fully comprehending the impact of jaundice in the severely ill infant.

It is not the intention of this chapter to discuss the in-depth use of reflexology for preterm and ill neonates, but reflex zone therapy undertaken by appropriately qualified neonatal nurses may be more freely available in the future. Integration of any complementary therapy into the care of such vulnerable infants can only succeed when there is more good-quality research regarding its effects, together with a greater understanding of the therapy amongst conventional neonatal practitioners.

STRESS FACTORS IN THE NEONATAL UNIT

Parents of babies in the neonatal intensive care unit experience many stressful emotions, including extreme anxiety, guilt, anger, fear and grief for the normal baby they have not been able to produce. They feel out of control and at the mercy of the medical and neonatal nursing staff and will almost certainly need to remain in the distressing environment of the hospital (Fig. 11-1, Plate 13) for longer than they would have originally envisaged. This can affect the mother physically, emotionally and spiritually, often contributing to the reduction of lactation either directly (perhaps because she is not eating sufficiently) or indirectly as a result of a compromised let-down reflex due to separation from the baby. Parents often feel a sense of failure, helplessness and negative self-regard at this difficult time in their lives (Griffin et al 1998) and providing a reflexology service for par-

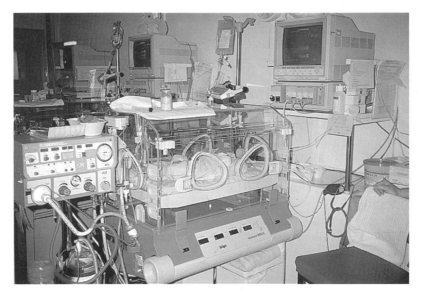

Figure 11.1   General view of a neonatal unit (see also Plate 13).

ents in the unit may assist in redressing these imbalances, helping parents to cope both physically and mentally.

Non-specific reflexology treatment acts as a relaxation for the mother, helping her to feel better about herself and giving confidence and empowerment. Gibson (1991) states that it is easier to understand empowerment when it is absent, giving examples of powerlessness, dependency, helplessness, hopelessness and a loss of control over life. These are all feelings and emotions that parents may feel at some time when they have a sick baby. Fathers particularly may have feelings of helplessness related to anxiety, caused by alterations in the parenting role (Miles et al 1992). Teaching fathers reflexology techniques to use on their partner helps them to share in the process of caring for their babies. Teaching both parents some simple reflexology techniques to perform on each other allows them to give mutual support and to assert some control over a situation where they are likely to feel out of control. Reflexology provided by neonatal unit staff has the added benefit of offering parents an opportunity to discuss their baby's progress in a more informal setting and to ask questions that at other times they might feel inhibited to ask. It is for this reason that reflexology practitioners who are not trained neonatal nurses or midwives will need to have a thorough understanding of the processes of adaptation and survival to which the baby is subject. It is inappropriate for lay practitioners to attempt to advise or counsel parents in these situations without adequate knowledge, training and authority.

Separation is another stress factor for the parents, particularly the mother, and this is exacerbated if the baby has been transferred to another neonatal unit for more specialized care. There is anecdotal evidence in these cases that the psychological effects of the separation are so great that the mother will request early discharge from hospital, putting her own health at risk, so that she can be with her baby (Griffin et al 1998).

The physical appearance and condition of the preterm or very ill infant is particularly difficult for parents to accept (Shields-Poe & Pinelli 1997). A mother's instinct is to cuddle and nurse her baby, yet she finds herself in a position where she perceives her child as so fragile that she is apprehensive to approach and touch (Perehudoff 1990). Although reflexology cannot change the situation, it can help the mother to achieve a more positive outlook.

The need to visit the baby daily in hospital, especially once the mother has been discharged, can be time-consuming and exhausting and may contribute to a temporary decrease in lactation (Griffin et al 1998, Lang 1997). These problems can be compounded by geographical distance, financial resources or other commitments such as other children. Providing reflexology treatments in the neonatal unit can be a welcome and beneficial service that enables mothers to recoup their energy prior to feeding their babies and to acknowledge the need for care of the whole family unit, not just the infant.

Shields-Poe & Pinelli (1997) debated the impact of the environment of the neonatal special or intensive care unit on parents. The unit may be busy,

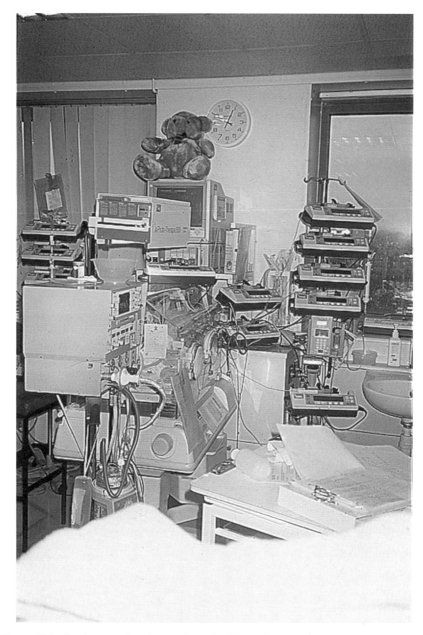

Figure 11.2 Incubator and equipment (see also Plate 14).

noisy and at first appear impersonal. The initial sight of their baby attached to a range of flashing monitors and life-support equipment can be daunting in the extreme and leave parents feeling exposed and vulnerable (Fig. 11.2, Plate 14) (Ingham et al 1994). The sounding of alarms on monitoring equipment can be particularly stressful, especially if they are due to mechanical malfunction (Miles 1989, cited in Griffin et al 1998).

Parents need to be given the opportunity to verbalize their concerns (Perehudoff 1990) and a reflexology session gives the mother an opportunity for individual attention in a quiet environment with time and space to voice any worries and concerns, enhancing relaxation and decreasing anxiety. Mothers can feel particularly disillusioned with the alteration in their parenting role (Miles et al 1992, Perehudoff 1990) and experience feelings of inadequacy at being unable to meet even the basic needs of their sick infants (Hayes et al 1993), leading to feelings of hopelessness and a desperate need to be valued (Griffin et al 1998). Reflexology may go some way towards reducing these feelings.

BREASTFEEDING IN THE NEONATAL UNIT

Breastfeeding and the provision of breast milk is the one activity that belongs solely to the mother. It is an emotionally significant and unique contribution to the infant's wellbeing (Kavanagh et al 1997). Jaeger et al (1997) state that, given informed choice, a mother would choose to breastfeed her sick infant in the knowledge that she was doing the best for her baby. However, although the nutritional, immunological and psychological advantages to the baby are well documented, Tureanu & Tureanu (1994) state that establishing and maintaining lactation, and the practicalities of breastfeeding in the neonatal setting, are incredibly difficult. Quite apart

---

Case study 11.1 Maggie

Although only 22, Maggie had suffered two miscarriages, which had caused her considerable emotional distress. The birth of her third child, Ellie, now 4, had also been traumatic. Consequently, when Adam was born at 25 weeks gestation by Caesarean section, it left Maggie feeling very frightened and vulnerable, and almost 'too scared to love him'.

Adam was nursed on the special care baby unit in an incubator and ventilated from birth. Maggie had great difficulty establishing lactation; there was an initial delay because of the Caesarean section and the use of postoperative drugs. However, by day 3, Maggie was using reflexology techniques and massaging her breasts prior to using the breast pump. Although lactation was slow, she was achieving between 20 and 30 ml daily, which gradually increased over the next week to up to 100 ml daily. This gave Adam a good start when he was well enough to commence milk feeds. However, by week 4 Maggie made the decision to stop lactation because her breasts were sore and she was only expressing very small amounts despite the use of reflexology techniques and being prescribed metoclopramide. Another factor that may have reduced lactation was separation and tiredness after her discharge home.

Maggie continued to receive reflexology at home, which helped her to relax and to feel secure enough to talk about her feelings for both the babies who had died and for Adam. She felt frightened of becoming too close to Adam in case he also died, these intense emotions may have contributed to adversely affecting her lactation.

from the physical advantages to the mother, breastfeeding provides an emotional and psychological link with the baby, helping to develop the mother–infant relationship, which may otherwise be inhibited by separation (Jones 1994).

Mothers of babies in the special or intensive care unit often struggle to initiate and maintain lactation because their babies are usually very small and sick, requiring mechanical ventilation and intensive care for weeks and perhaps even months. It might be impossible for the mother to breastfeed her baby physically if the baby is receiving mechanical ventilation or requires reverse barrier nursing care (Case study 11.1). If the baby is extremely preterm then the physiological changes that occur in the last few weeks of a full-term pregnancy to prepare the mother for lactation will not

---

Case study 11.2 Jane

Jane had a normal term delivery of a healthy baby boy. Four days after delivery Jane's breasts remained soft and lactation seemed very slow to become established. Reflexology was performed by the midwife–reflexologist in the maternity unit, with treatment focusing on the zones for the pituitary gland, to stimulate oxytocin production, and on the breast zones. Within 5 minutes, Jane experienced hardening of the breasts and the commencement of lactation. Even the midwife–reflexologist could not believe the speed of the response!

It is probable that Jane was particularly sensitive to reflexology because her responses were so immediate and so dramatic. It might simply have been the relaxation effect that assisted Jane's own let down reflex, but is more likely to have been this in combination with a physiological impact of the treatment.

Case study 11.3 Kay

Kay's first baby, Mandy, was born prematurely at 25 weeks gestation and transferred to the special care baby unit because she required intensive care, with ventilation and incubation.

Kay started expressing breast milk for Mandy from day 2 and although the supply was slow to start, it was becoming well established by day 4. In accordance with normal practice, the expressed milk was frozen and stored until Mandy needed it. However, by day 14 the amount of milk Kay was able to express on each occasion had decreased to 30 ml and she became increasingly despondent. Metoclopramide produced no real improvement and it was decided to try reflexology, working on the points for the pituitary gland, breast areas and solar plexus. Within 2 days, Kay's milk supply had increased to 100 ml expressed on each occasion, which could have been partly attributed to the reflexology.

However, the treatment may have assisted in a more indirect way. Mandy's condition had been very unstable but by the time of Kay's reflexology she had been off the ventilator for 3 days and nursed on continuous positive airways pressure, which is much less invasive and is perceived by parents as major progress in the baby's recovery. Since Mandy had been born, Kay had felt unable to leave her, wanting to spend as much time as possible with her daughter. After the reflexology Kay felt able to leave Mandy overnight, starting a longer term change in her mothering role and it may be that the treatment gave Kay the confidence to leave Mandy once she began to improve.

have taken place. In addition, the health of the mother may have been a reason for the early or traumatic birth of the baby and the mother may continue to be unwell for some time, for example, with acute pregnancy-induced hypertension, severe anaemia following haemorrhage or recovering from Caesarean section. The effort required to express breast milk for administration to the baby via a nasogastric tube can be physically and emotionally draining, eventually leading to a dramatic reduction in the amount of milk produced, although expressing breast milk and leaving it on the special care baby unit has profound importance for the mother because it provides a connection with her baby even when she cannot be there (Kavanagh et al 1997).

The majority of lactation problems associated specifically with feeding preterm and very sick babies appear to be stress related (Case study 11.3). A search by this author revealed no specific literature or research evidence concerning the use of reflexology to aid lactation by physiologically stimulating oxytocin output, although Tiran (1996) suggests that there is much anecdotal evidence for effectiveness in increasing milk production (Case study 11.2). However, although there is a need for both qualitative and quantitative research to substantiate the evidence in this respect, reflexology research findings on the effects on emotional and psychological wellbeing can be applied to mothers whose inadequate lactation appears to be exacerbated by emotional stress. For example, Trousdell (1996) found that patients with mental health problems responded positively to reflexology treatments with increased self-esteem, confidence, motivation and concentration and reported valuing the 'time for self' and the opportunity to talk to the therapist. In many women these indirect results may be sufficient to induce an improved sense of wellbeing that contributes to a more efficient lactation process.

Maternal fear and anxiety induce a physiological stress response that results in the release of adrenaline. Adrenaline affects lactation by suppressing the release of the oxytocin required to produce breast milk (Jaeger et al 1997, Simpoulas et al 1995). Reflexology may assist in reducing the intensity of these feelings by restoring homeostasis in mind and spirit, and thus in the body. Working specific reflexes in the feet or hands brings about a sense of relaxation, which in turn improves circulation and transportation of the required elements to repair and balance the whole, allowing hormonal equilibrium to occur (Kunz & Kunz 1999).

Brendstrup et al (1997) successfully determined that reflexology treated migraine and tension headaches without the side-effects of using drugs and Dryden et al (1999) reported statistically significant reductions in systolic blood pressure following reflexology (albeit with a small sample size of 19). Stress in mothers with babies in the neonatal unit may manifest with headaches, migraines or a prolongation of the hypertension that might have been a reason for an induced preterm delivery, so it seems logical to consider the use of reflexology to reduce the physical implications of these stressors.

The mode of delivery, notably Caesarean section, can have an impact on the baby. Maternal anaesthesia and analgesia have various effects on the fetus, often resulting in a lethargic baby with a poor sucking reflex, which can result in a delay in the establishment of lactation (Matthews 1988). A very preterm baby will also have an underdeveloped sucking reflex and, if the mother has had a general anaesthetic, she may be too sick or sleepy to use a breast pump properly for the first 24 hours after delivery. It is interesting to note that the reflexology points for the breasts situated on the hand lie in the area that might have been the site for an intravenous infusion cannula and some reflexologists believe that this, or severe bruising caused by an interstitial infusion in the back of the hand, can inhibit lactation on that side. Other complementary therapies, such as homeopathic arnica, may need to be used for relief of the bruising but, on resolution, mothers could be advised to massage this area of the hand to increase stimulation of the breasts.

CONCLUSION

This chapter has explored the potential of reflexology for parents whose babies are admitted to the neonatal special and intensive care unit. The administration of reflexology to preterm and severely ill neonates is not advocated unless the practitioner is a neonatal nurse and an experienced reflex zone therapist. The discussion has, however, raised many questions, highlighting the need for research to confirm or refute the anecdotal evidence in relation to the use of reflexology for neonates and its effects on lactation in the mothers of these infants. Teaching reflexology techniques to parents can empower them and contribute to an improved sense of control and to greater wellbeing. Provision of a reflexology service within the neonatal unit offers parents an opportunity to relax and to discuss their worries and concerns about their baby's progress.

REFERENCES

Acolet D, Modi N, Giannakoulopoulos X et al. Changes in plasma cortisol and catecholamine concentrations in response to massage in preterm infants. Archives of Disease in Childhood (Fetal and Neonatal Edition) 1993; 68(1):29–31.
Adamson-Macedo EN, Dattani I, Wilson A et al. Small sample follow up study of children who received tactile stimulation after preterm birth: intelligence and achievements. Journal of Reproductive and Infant Psychology 1993; 11(3):165–168.
Adamson-Macedo EN, De Roiste A, Wilson A et al. TAC-TIC therapy with high risk distressed ventilated preterms. Journal of Reproductive and Infant Psychology 1994a; 12(4):249–252.
Adamson-Macedo EN, Attree JLA, Wilson A et al. TAC-TIC therapy : the importance of systematic stroking. British Journal of Midwifery 1994b; 2(6):264, 266–269.

Adamson-Macedo EN, De Roiste A, Wilson A et al. Systematic gentle/light stroking and maternal random touching of ventilated preterms: a preliminary study. International Journal of Perinatal Psychology and Medicine 1997; 9(1):17–31.

Brendstrup E, Launso L, Eriksen L. Headaches and reflexological treatment. In: Association of Reflexologists. Reflexology Research Reports. 4th edn. London: Association of Reflexologists; 1997.

De Roiste A, Bushnell IWR. The immediate gastric effects of a tactile stimulation programme on premature infants. Journal of Reproductive and Infant Psychology 1995; 13(1):57–62.

De Roiste A, Bushnell I, Burns J. TAC-TIC: how do special care baby unit babies react to it? British Journal of Midwifery 1995; 3(1):8–10, 12–15.

Dryden SL, Holden SA, Mackereth PA. 'Just the ticket': the findings of a pilot complementary therapy service (part II). Complementary Therapies in Nursing and Midwifery 1999; 5:15–18.

Field T, Schanburg SM, Scafidi F et al. Tactile/kinesthetic stimulation effects on preterm neonates. Pediatrics 1986; 77(5):654–658.

Griffin T, Wishba C, Kavanagh K. Nursing interventions to reduce stress in parents of hospitalized preterm infants. Journal of Pediatric Nursing 1998; 13(5):290–295.

Harrison LL, Leeper JD, Yoon M. Effects of early parent touch on preterm infants' heart rates and arterial oxygen saturation levels. Journal of Advanced Nursing 1990; 15(8):877–885.

Hayes N, Stainton MC, McNeil D. Caring for a chronically ill infant: a paradigm case of maternal rehearsal in the neonatal intensive care unit. Journal of Pediatric Nursing 1993; 8(6):355–360.

Helders PJM, Cats BP, Van Der Net J et al. The effects of a tactile stimulation/range-finding programme on the development of very low birth weight infants during initial hospitalisation. Child Care, Health and Development 1988; 14(5):341–353.

Ingham J, Redshaw M, Harris A. Breastfeeding in neonatal care. British Journal of Midwifery 1994; 2(9):412–418.

Jaeger MC, Lawson M, Filteau S. The impact of prematurity and neonatal illness on the decision to breast-feed. Journal of Advanced Nursing 1997; 25:729–737.

Jones E. Breast feeding the pre-born infant. Modern Midwife 1994; January:22–26.

Kavanagh K, Meier P, Zimmerman B, Mead L. The rewards outweigh the efforts: breastfeeding outcomes mothers of preterm infants. Journal of Human Lactation 1997; 13(1):15–21.

Kuhn CM, Schanberg SM, Filed T et al. Tactile-kinesthetic stimulation effects on sympathetic and adrenocorticol function in preterm infants. Journal of Pediatrics 1991; 119(3):434–440.

Kunz K, Kunz B. The complete guide to foot reflexology. Self-published: Albuquerque, New Mexico; 1993.

Lang S. Breastfeeding special case babies. London: Baillière Tindall; 1997.

Lett A. Reflex zone therapy for health professionals. Edinburgh: Churchill Livingstone; 2000.

Matthews MK. The relationship between maternal labour analgesia and delay in the initiation of breastfeeding in healthy neonates in the early neonatal period. Midwifery 1988; 5:3–10.

Miles MS. Parents of chronically ill premature infants: sources of stress. Critical Care Nursing Quarterly 1989; 12(3):69–74. Cited in: Griffin T, Wishba C, Kavanagh K. Nursing interventions to reduce stress in parents of hospitalised preterm infants. Journal of Paediatric Nursing 1998; 13(5):290–297.

Miles MS, Funk SG, Kasper MA. The stress response of mothers and fathers of preterm infants. Research in Nursing and Health 1992; 15:261–269.

Perehudoff B. Parents perceptions of environmental stressors in the special care nursery. Neonatal Network 1990; 9(2):29–44.

Shields-Poe D, Pinelli J. Variables associated with parental stress in neonatal intensive care units. Neonatal Network 1997; 16(1):29–37.

Simpoulas AP, Dutra de Oliveira JE, Desai ID, eds. Behavioral and metabolic aspects of breastfeeding: international trends. Basel, Switzerland: Karger; 1995.

Tiran D. The use of complementary therapies in midwifery practice: a focus on reflexology. Complementary Therapies in Nursing and Midwifery 1996; 2:32–37.

Trousdell P. Reflexology meets emotional needs. International Journal of Alternative and Complementary Medicine 1996; November:9–12.

Tureanu L, Tureanu V. A clinical evaluation of the effectiveness of acupuncture for insufficient lactation. American Journal of Acupuncture 1994; 22(1):23–27.

Walker P. Baby massage. London: Piatkus; 1995.

White-Traut RC, Nelson MN. Maternally administered tactile, auditory, visual and vestibular stimulation: relationship to later interactions between mothers and premature infants. Research in Nursing and Health 1988; 11:31–39.

FURTHER READING

Achterberg J. Imagery in healing shamanism and modern medicine. London: Shambala; 1985.

Affonso DD, Hurst IL, Mayberry LH et al. Stressors reported by mothers of hospitalized premature infants. Neonatal Network 1992; 11(60):63–70.

Akre J. Infant feeding the physiological basis. Geneva: World Health Organization; 1990.

Clavey S. The use of acupuncture for the treatment of insufficient lactation. American Journal of Acupuncture 1996; 24(1):35–46.

Ehrenkranz RA, Ackerman BA. Metoclopramide effect on faltering milk production by mothers of premature infants. Paediatrics 1986; 78(4):614–620.

Gibson CH. A concept analysis of empowerment. Journal of Advanced Nursing 1991; 16:354–361.

Harris PE. Acupressure: a review of the literature. Complementary Therapies in Medicine 1997; 5(3):156–161.

Ingham J, Redshaw M, Harris A. Breastfeeding in neonatal care. British Journal of Midwifery 1994; 2(9):412–418.

Jaeger MC, Lawson M, Filteau S. The impact of prematurity and neonatal illness on the decision to breast-feed. Journal of Advanced Nursing 1997; 25:729–737.

Johanson RB, Spencer SA, Rolfe P et al. Effect of post-delivery care on neonatal body temperature. Acta Paediatrica 1992; 81(11):859–863.

Rankin-Box D. Innovations in practice: complementary therapies in nursing. Complementary Therapies in Medicine 1993; 1:30–33.

Rankin-Box D. Therapies in practice: a survey assessing nurses' use of complementary therapies. Complementary Therapies in Nursing and Midwifery 1997; 3:92–99.

Shields-Poe D, Pinelli J. Variables associated with parental stress in neonatal intensive care units. Neonatal Network 1997; 16(1):29–37.

Simpoulas AP, Dutra de Oliveira JE, Desai ID, eds. Behavioral and metabolic aspects of breastfeeding: international trends. Basel, Switzerland: Karger; 1995.

Smith P. Research mindedness for practice – an interactive approach for nursing and health care. Edinburgh: Churchill Livingstone; 1997.

Tipping L, Mackereth PA. A concept analysis: the effect of reflexology on homeostasis to establish and maintain lactation. Complementary Therapies in Nursing and Midwifery 2000; 6:189–198.

West Z. Acupuncture within the national health service: a personal perspective. Complementary Therapies in Nursing and Midwifery 1997; 3:83–86.

12

Advocating the use of reflexology for people with a learning disability

Evelyn Gale

Touch and reflexology
Indications for the use of reflexology
    for people with learning disabilities
Reflexology and Snoezelen
Informed consent
A reflexology code of practice for
    working with people with learning
    disabilities

Conclusion
References
Further reading
Useful addresses

Abstract

This chapter explores the value of reflexology for people with a learning disability, including its use within a Snoezelen environment. Other issues pertinent to the practice of reflexology specifically with this client group are also considered.

Key words: learning disability, touch, consent, normalization, Snoezelen

People with a learning disability are usually diagnosed at or shortly after birth. Their disability is usually chronic, lasting throughout their lifetime and making them amongst the most vulnerable and socially excluded in our society; they are frequently under valued and ill served (Matson & Mulick, 1983). The term 'learning disability' is used in the UK to describe people with significant developmental delay that results in arrested or incomplete achievement of the 'normal' milestones of human development (Gates & Beacock 1997). There are about 210 000 people with severe learning disabilities in England and about 1.2 million with a mild or moderate learning disability (DoH 2001).

Communication between health professionals and clients is usually primarily verbal. Questions are asked and answers sought by both practitioner and client in an attempt to determine the most appropriate course of treatment or management of the presenting condition. Even children are normally able to assist in this process, with support from their parent or guardian. In reflexology practice verbal communication is used in conjunction with other interpersonal skills to support the therapeutic relationship

(Mackereth 1999). Often the client will talk to, and be listened to, by the therapist. The therapist's willingness to listen, and their use of 'quality time', is conducive to developing the therapeutic relationship, and to influencing the client's responses (Wall & Wheeler 1996). Similarly, the practitioner uses verbal communication to impart information to the client, that may empower them to act in partnership with the therapist, for example, by implementing lifestyle changes. However, a major difficulty in working with people with severe learning disabilities is that they may have few or limited verbal skills, potentially preventing them from benefiting fully from a therapy that is partly dependent on verbal communication. Nonverbal ways of developing a therapeutic relationship are therefore essential, with touch being one of the most important.

TOUCH AND REFLEXOLOGY

'Touching' can be interpreted as the acknowledgement of a person's presence, a display of love, an act of aggression, a desire for comfort or a feeling of closeness (Gale & Hegarty 2000). Touching is an intimate act, be it a simple handshake or a tender embrace, with the potential for a relationship to develop. Reflexology provides *quality* touch for clients and an opportunity for the practitioner to identify non-verbal cues and respond to a client's individual needs. When used as part of a care plan by learning disability carers it may become a sharing and empowering process, enabling both client and practitioner to benefit as the relationship develops and communication is stimulated and enhanced. For people with severe or profound learning disabilities, the touch of reflexology can be a vitally important primary sense if they are unable to communicate through more conventional channels (Gates 1997).

For people with a learning disability, touch may be experienced in mainly functional ways, such as in feeding or bathing, which may be perceived as affirmative and supportive but may also be felt to be coarse and manipulating. For such people, touch that has a more therapeutic focus may be rare, perhaps because of a natural reluctance of people to relate adequately to those who are 'different' from the socially acceptable norm. Gale & Hegarty (2000) explored the use of touch for adults with severe to profound learning disability in a non-participant, observational study of the work routines of carers in three different residential care settings. The results showed that clients received more 'functional' touch, primarily to the hands, (purposeful touching to help with everyday functions) than 'expressive' or 'therapeutic' touch. 'Expressive' touch is the act of touching a person spontaneously with emotional intent to express feelings; 'therapeutic' touch aims to benefit the person either physically or psychologically. Clients reacted with more positive non-verbal responses when expressive or therapeutic touch was used, whereas functional touch elicited negative responses such as aggression and inhibition.

Unfortunately, work by Wolfensberger (1972) in the 1970s all but eliminated the use of expressive touch with people with learning disabilities. Healthcare practitioners came to believe that it was not a 'culturally normative activity' and activities such as indiscriminate hugging were viewed as de-valuing the client and perpetuating the 'permanent child'. More recently, this view has changed; reflexology and other bodywork therapies such as massage offer an appropriate and valued means of touch, providing valuable physical and emotional contact.

Cohen (1987) reported the use of the metamorphic technique on a 24-year-old deaf and blind man with learning disability, initiating the relationship without touching him but enabling him to absorb her presence. Once he had become accustomed to her smell and touch he would communicate to her the places he wished to be touched by moving her hands to the appropriate place and by smiling. Although a slow process, this interaction enabled the client to become relaxed and happy and to improve his communication skills and concentration whilst reducing his behavioural problems.

Similarly, Gray (1990) recounted the experience of working with a young woman with a severe learning disability involving extreme disruptive and self-injurious behaviour who responded to regular reflexology with a reduction in head banging, notable relaxation, increased smiling and becoming more sociable. These examples demonstrate a potentiality in the care of people with learning disabilities that may, as yet, not be fully recognized. The importance of using appropriate touch in the provision of care of people with a learning disability is limited to only a few published papers and these are mainly impressionistic and anecdotal, although such evidence should not be discounted completely. Indeed, Sanderson et al (1991) have extensive experience of using massage and aromatherapy with clients with learning disability.

INDICATIONS FOR THE USE OF REFLEXOLOGY FOR PEOPLE WITH LEARNING DISABILITIES

Reflexology is a non-invasive, cost-effective therapy requiring no equipment yet producing powerful responses in recipients. It has an advantage over body massage in that only the feet need to be accessible, or the hands, eliminating the need to undress. It can be performed in any setting and does not necessarily require a separate treatment room if the person prefers to remain with others. This has particular benefits for people with learning disabilities living in residential accommodation who may be disturbed by others entering the room inadvertently.

When performed by professionals such as nurses or social workers already caring for the client, reflexology will strengthen the relationship and may produce other advantages to the overall care of the individual. Additional time will be required if an independent practitioner is to establish a therapeutic relationship with each client, and this is less cost effective and may be more disruptive than reflexology that is performed by existing carers. Relatives could be taught simple reflexology strategies to perform when they visit, which may assist situations where the intermittent arrival and departure of a close relative triggers behavioural or mood changes.

The use of reflexology in helping people with challenging behaviours such as aggression, destruction or self-injury may be of benefit along with more conventional treatments including structured activities, applied behaviour analysis and sensory integrative approaches. Exhibiting challenging behaviour may be the only means of communicating anxiety and stress (Hegarty & Gale 1996) and reflexology may help to reduce this by inducing deep relaxation (Booth 1994, Griffiths 2001). The need for night sedation may be reduced by the relaxation effect aiding sleep of increased quality and duration, and was reported as an outcome for patients in a study by Dryden et al (1999). Hyperactivity may also be reduced leading to more socially acceptable behaviour. The sense of relaxation may engender an appreciation of sensual pleasure which may have been denied to people with a learning disability, enhancing their subconscious sense of self-worth and decreasing self-injurious behaviour. Regular reflexology provides something to which they can look forward and an additional activity in a life where variety may be limited.

Up to 30% of people with a severe learning disability have additional sensory or physical impairments (Sines 1992), up to 7 in 10 people with severe learning disabilities have measurable hearing loss and more than 7 in 10 suffer from sight problems (Thompson 1993); this is a far greater prevalence than in the general population. Reflexology may help to improve general health, revitalizing people physically, emotionally and spiritually and helping to enhance quality of life. The effects of immobility for those with a physical as well as a learning disability who are confined to a wheelchair may be relieved by reflexology through the circulatory improvements that are thought to occur (Dryden et al 1999). Hand reflexology may be necessary for someone with major lower limb impairments although gentle, short episodes of foot reflexology over a protracted period of time may eventually help to improve mobility and reduce pain. Stimulation of the excretory processes to reduce constipation arising from immobility may decrease the use of regular laxatives (Joyce & Richardson 1997). Those whose head banging causes headaches (which may lead to further aggressive behaviour) may find that the symptom can be relieved through reflexology (Lafuente et al 1997). The emotional frustration, anger, tension and discomfort which is apparent in many women with learning disability prior to menstruation may also respond well to the relaxing effects of reflexology, which at the same time encourages physiological processes to normalize, thereby possibly reducing breast tenderness, abdominal bloating and regulating the cycle. A study by O'Dwyer et al (1995) investigated the contribution of menstruation to the occurrence of aggressive incidents over a 2-year period in women with a learning disability. The results suggested that there was no significant increase in aggressive incidents before or during menstruation, but that those with primary amenorrhoea had significantly higher rates of aggressive incidents.

The Department of Health (1995) focused attention on the health needs of people with learning disability, emphasizing the importance of health surveillance, access, promotion and prevention. Reflexology may serve as a preventive healthcare strategy, for example by strengthening the immune system (Griffiths 2001) or reducing blood pressure (Frankel 1997). Regular treatment by the same therapist may lead to improved identification of impending physical health problems, for example, urinary tract infection, both through the continuity of care and through the diagnostic potential of the therapy (see Chapter 3), facilitating more rapid treatment and reducing the risk of complications.

REFLEXOLOGY AND SNOEZELEN

A popular therapeutic approach for people with learning disability is sensory stimulation by means of 'Snoezelen' (the word is derived from the Dutch for 'doze' and 'smell'). Snoezelen (Figs 12.1 and 12.2, Plates 15 and 16)

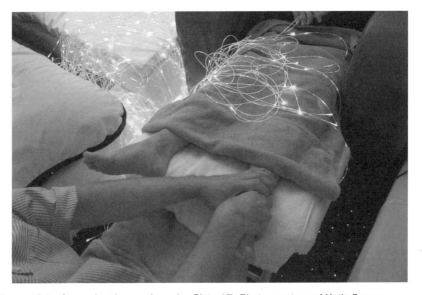

Figure 12.1   Snoezelen therapy (see also Plate 15). Photo courtesy of Katie Spruce BA (Hons), medical photographer, Christie Hospital NHS Trust, with permission.

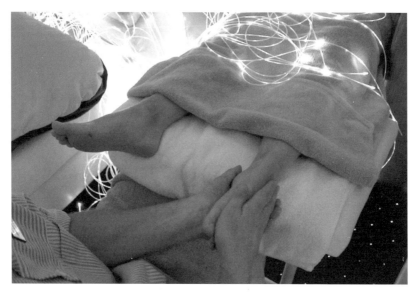

Figure 12.2 Snoezelen therapy (see also Plate 16). Photo courtesy of Katie Spruce BA (Hons), medical photographer, Christie Hospital NHS Trust, with permission.

is based on the belief that people with profound learning disabilities interact with the environment primarily through sensory and motor stimulation of sight, hearing, touch, smell and taste (Cunningham et al 1991, Hutchinson 1994). The process involves the use of a specially adapted sensory room together with an 'enabling' non-directive approach to therapy (Hutchinson 1991). This stimulation invokes environmental manipulation to effect internal change in the client, decreasing maladaptive behaviours and reducing stress (King 1993). Touch, usually in the form of non-invasive contact by holding or stroking the hands and feet is valuable and reflexology could similarly be used within the Snoezelen environment, potentially relieving stress and anxiety to encourage a sense of psychological wellbeing, and also facilitating homeostasis. It will also foster a therapeutic relationship through enhanced communication, thus empowering the client and enabling them to feel respected and valued.

Many Snoezelen and therapy rooms for people with learning disabilities utilize aromatherapy essential oils to stimulate the sense of smell and develop an affinity to particular pleasant aromas (Armstrong & Heidingsfeld 2000) and, although many reflexologists prefer not to mix therapies, this may be a situation in which a combination of reflexology with aromatherapy foot massage could work synergistically to the benefit of the client. Siting the reflexology treatments within the Snoezelen room may also emphasize its therapeutic value and enable clients to focus fully on its sensory impact (Case study 12.1).

Case study 12.1   Daniel

Daniel was a 32-year-old man with a severe learning disability and additional sensory impairments. Nurses caring for him in the residential centre believed that he benefited from Snoezelen therapy. After a few sessions he would immediately remove his socks and shoes on entering the room, indicating that he wanted his feet to be massaged and one of the nurses would perform a 20-minute foot massage incorporating reflexology strokes. Daniel obviously enjoyed this and demonstrated his pleasure by smiling and laughing. After a short period of time he would begin to relax and eventually fall asleep. This was the only activity in which Daniel would engage whilst in the Snoezelen room.

INFORMED CONSENT

Quality care requires individual attention and respect, a personal sense of commitment and a degree of responsibility (Basford 1995). Using care is an art that requires commitment, knowledge and encompasses a feeling of dedication to another. The practice of reflexology must take account of the same standards and ethical considerations as any other therapeutic practice. However, one major consideration in the use of reflexology with people with learning disabilities is the complex issue of informed consent. Issues to consider are the differences between approval and objection, the way a person communicates, and the time in which a person has the opportunity to give consent. It is important to note that fear, force or fraud can undermine consent (Gates 1997). A number of competing interests need to be taken into account in any review of the legal issues in this area. On the client's side of the relationship there may be tension between maximizing freedom and autonomy and ensuring that the client receives appropriate treatment (DoH 1995). On the professional's side, that the practitioner must have the freedom to make appropriate clinical decisions, confident of being within the limits of good practice but also having the protection of the law (Hillery et al 1998). In the case of people who seem less capable of understanding their own needs and the consequences of decisions made concerning them, these tensions are heightened. It is essential that the client understands the nature of the therapy, but this may take time to explain or demonstrate. Verbal and non-verbal cues must be recognized and interpreted correctly and the client may also need the support of an independent advocate in making decisions. A method must be developed to ensure that people who cannot give consent are protected (i.e. in their right to treatment and their right to autonomy) and also ensure that professionals feel secure in their clinical activities with this client group.

A REFLEXOLOGY CODE OF PRACTICE FOR WORKING WITH PEOPLE WITH LEARNING DISABILITIES

The vulnerability of people with learning disabilities and their status within our society leaves them open to abuse, albeit unintentional in many cases. Whilst reflexology is performed with positive intent to heal the body, mind and spirit, it is possible that boundaries may inadvertently be transgressed unless care is taken to avoid this. Many people with learning disabilities are cared for in a range of institutional settings and increasingly reflexology is one of the therapeutic strategies on offer. However, all practitioners, whether already working in a caring capacity with these clients or visiting as an independent practitioner, should adhere to a set of guidelines for ethical and quality practice. The following guidelines relate equally to the care of people other than those with learning disabilities but can be applied specifically to this client group, and are suggestions for good practice.

- The practitioner must be adequately and appropriately trained and experienced to practise reflexology in a learning disability setting, including a comprehensive understanding of specific elements of learning disability and their physiopathological, psychosocial and spiritual impacts on individuals; where possible this should be based on available evidence for its safety and efficacy.
- Reflexology should be structured into the care plans for individuals, in collaboration with the multidisciplinary professional team.
- The client must be offered a choice, presented in a way which they are able to understand, in order that they can give consent to receiving reflexology in as informed a way as possible.
- The setting for the reflexology should be conducive to a therapeutic environment and all aspects of the client's health, safety and overall wellbeing should be addressed.
- The development of a working relationship between the practitioner and the client will be dependent on assessing the needs of the individual, taking into account aspects such as mood or behavioural changes which may influence the relationship.
- Not all clients will be receptive to touch and it is as important to identify those for whom reflexology may not be appropriate.
- Verbal and non-verbal cues must be recognized and interpreted correctly.
- Comprehensive and contemporaneous records of reflexology treatment must be maintained.
- Practitioners will need to acknowledge their own feelings towards touching clients with learning disabilities and may require opportunities to discuss them with other professionals through clinical supervision (Mackereth 2000).

CONCLUSION

The needs of individuals for physical contact vary enormously and the practitioner should therefore evaluate a client's responses towards the interaction taking place when touched through reflexology and recognize the ways in which the client might interpret that interaction. The type of touch used may affect the client's physical, psychological, social and spiritual needs, with expressive and therapeutic touch having a more positively significant effect on the therapeutic relationship than functional touch. Reflexology should be incorporated into the type of care that is central to valuing people with a learning disability. It offers a therapeutic intervention which affects the person physically, emotionally and spiritually, enhancing their self-esteem, relaxing through sensual appreciation and empowering by effecting changes in overall health and wellbeing.

Reflexology is increasingly and enthusiastically being introduced into the care of people with learning disabilities and provides a valuable therapeutic tool. The principles inherent in anecdotal accounts of reflexology practice by nurses in hospitals (Barron 1990, Crowther 1991, Lockett 1992) and by midwives (Tiran 1996) can be applied to the field of learning disability, but more contemporary and related investigations are needed as the amount of published research specifically related to this client group is very limited. Reflexologists have an obligation to ensure that their practice is of the highest possible standard, safe, cost-effective, based on all available evidence and efficacious for predetermined outcomes. Guidelines for ethical practice may be helpful in ensuring that these obligations are met.

REFERENCES

Armstrong F, Heidingsfeld V. Aromatherapy for deaf and deaf blind people living in residential accommodation. Complementary Therapies in Nursing and Midwifery 2000; 6:180–188.
Barron H. Towards better health with reflexology. Nursing Standard 1990; 4(40):32–33.
Basford L. Professional care. The theory and practice of nursing. An integrated approach to patient care. London: Capion Press Ltd; 1995.
Booth B. Reflexology. Nursing Times 1994; 90(1):38–40.
Cohen N. Massage is the message. Nursing Times 1987; 83(19):19–20.
Crowther D. Complementary therapies in practice. Nursing Standard 1991; 5(23):25–27.
Cunningham CC, Hutchinson R, Kewin J. Recreation for people with profound and severe learning disabilities: The Whittington Hall 'Snoezelen' Project. Chesterfield: North Derbyshire Health Authority; 1991.
Department of Health (DoH). The health of the nation: a strategy for people with a learning disability. London: HMSO; 1995.
Department of Health (DoH). Valuing people: a new strategy for learning disability for the 21st century. London: HMSO; 2001.
Dryden S, Holden S, Mackereth P. 'Just the ticket'; the findings of a pilot complementary therapy service (Part II). Complementary Therapies in Nursing and Midwifery 1999; 5(1):15–18.
Frankel B. The effect of reflexology on barreceptor reflex sensitivity, blood pressure and sinus arrhythmia. Complementary Therapies in Medicine 1997; 5:80–84.
Gale E, Hegarty JR. The use of touch in caring for people with learning disability. The British Journal of Developmental Disabilities 2000; 46(2):97–108.
Gates B. Learning Disabilities. Edinburgh: Churchill Livingstone; 1997.

Gates B, Beacock C. Dimensions of learning disability London: Baillière Tindall; 1997.

Gray N. Healing by the laying on of hands. The Independent, January 2 1990.

Griffiths P. Reflexology. In: Rankin-Box D, ed. The nurse's handbook of complementary therapies. 2nd edn. London: Harcourt Publishers Ltd; 2001.

Hegarty JR, Gale E. Touch as a therapeutic medium for people with challenging behaviours. British Journal of Learning Disabilities 1996; 24:26–31.

Hillery J, Tomkin, D, McAuley A, et al. Consent to treatment and people with learning disabilities. Irish Journal of Psychological Medicine 1998; 15(4):117–118.

Hutchinson R. Sensory environments and experiences. Some ideas for application. In: Hutchinson R, Keewin J, eds. Sensation and disability. London: Rompa; 1991.

Joyce M, Richardson R. Reflexology can help MS. International Journal of Alternative and Complementary Medicine 1997; July: 10–12.

King BH. Self-injury by people with mental retardation: a compulsive behaviour hypothesis. American Journal of Mental Retardation 1993; 98:93–112.

Lafuente A, Nouera M, Puy C, et al. Effects of treatment with stimulation of the reflex zones of the foot with regard to the prophylactic Flunarizin™ treatment of patients suffering from headaches. In: Reflexology research reports. 4th edn. London: Association of Reflexologists; 1997: 39–40.

Lockett J. Reflexology – a nursing tool. The Australian Nurses Journal 1992; 22(1):14–15.

Mackereth PA. An introduction to catharsis and the healing crisis in reflexology. Complementary Therapies in Nursing and Midwifery 1999; 5(3):67–74.

Mackereth P. Clinical supervision. In: Rankin-Box D, ed. The Nurse's Handbook of Complementary Therapies. 2nd edn. London: Harcourt Publishers Ltd; 2000.

Matson JL, Mulick JC. Handbook of mental retardation. Washington DC: Pergamon Press; 1983.

O'Dwyer JM, Holmes J, Friedman T. Menstruation and aggression in a population of women with learning disabilities. British Journal of Learning Disabilities 1995; 23:51–55.

Sanderson H, Harrison J, Price S. Aromatherapy and massage for people with learning disability. Birmingham: Hands-on Publishing; 1991.

Sines D. Caring for people with learning disability (RCN Nursing update). Nursing Standard 1992; 25(7):3–8.

Thompson D. Learning disabilities the fundamental facts. London: The Mental Health Foundation; 1993.

Tiran D. The use of complementary therapies in midwifery practice: a focus on reflexology. Complementary Therapies in Nursing and Midwifery 1996; 2(2):32–37.

Wall M, Wheeler S. Benefits of the placebo effect in the therapeutic relationship. Complementary Therapies in Nursing and Midwifery 1996; 2(6):160–163.

Wolfensberger W. The principle of normalisation in human services. Toronto: National Institute on Mental Retardation 1972.

FURTHER READING

Davis PK. The power of Touch. Carson, Canada: Hay House Inc; 1991.

Sanderson H, Harrison J, Price S. Aromatherapy and massage for people with a learning disability. Birmingham: Hands-on Publishing; 1991.

USEFUL ADDRESSES

For details of equipment for Snoezelen rooms.
Rompa, Goytside Road, Chesterfield, Derbyshire, S41 0SW
Tel: 01246 211777
Fax: 01246 221802

Website: http://www.rompa.com/snoezelen.html
E-mail: enquiry@rompa.com.uk

Consent & Learning Disabilities
Department of Health website. Available: http://www.doh.gov.uk

13

Improving and maintaining mental health

Christine Knowles and Grace Higgins

The value of reflexology for people
  with mental health problems
Concerns, precautions and
  contraindications to reflexology
Working with people who have acute
  and/or enduring mental health
  problems

Ethical and legal concerns
Summary: a model of reflexology
  practice in mental health
Conclusion
References
Useful addresses

Abstract

This chapter explores the use of reflexology as a therapeutic intervention for those experiencing mental health problems such as stress, anxiety and depression, which may compromise their ability to cope with the pace and change of modern life.

Key words: anxiety, depression, stress, empowerment, safety, role boundaries

Everyone experiences stress at some time in their lives; indeed, mild stress is necessary to facilitate appropriate reactions to certain circumstances. However, some people are less able than others to deal with stressful life events, such as divorce, bereavement, moving home, redundancy and physical illness (Holmes & Rahe 1967). Ongoing stress can eventually accumulate and lead to a variety of physical symptoms and emotional problems such as weight loss, insomnia, anxiety, depression and behavioural changes (Donnellan 1997). If problems persist and interfere with activities of daily living it may result in an acute or chronic mental illness. This can be mild to extremely severe in terms of its effect on the person's ability to function cognitively and physically, be in relationships with others, cope with the challenges of life and find joy in their lives.

Mental illness can affect anyone, regardless of gender, social class, age or social support and as many as one in four may suffer depression at some point in their lives (Boseley 2001). It is also important to acknowledge that there remains a stigma attached to a diagnosis of mental illness, which can cause patients and their families to feel disenfranchised and isolated (Newell & Gournay 2000).

Mental illness can be brought on by many predisposing factors, which affect the biological, psychosocial and sociocultural aspects of a person's life. There may be a genetic tendency, which predisposes family members to mental ill health (Stuart & Sundeen 1995). Endocrine imbalances may affect behaviour and mood, as seen in people with hyperthyroidism in whom the elevated hormone levels can cause irritability, restlessness and anxiety. People with chronic pain, enduring ill health or disabilities may also experience a range of psychological difficulties in response to the situation they are in, often exacerbated by medication and side-effects, as well as other stresses or illnesses.

Disturbing life events can also exacerbate depression, anxiety, low self-esteem and confidence. This loss of self-esteem can result in an overwhelming feeling of helplessness and loss of control, which leads to negative thoughts and feelings sometimes resulting in suicidal tendencies, especially in young people (DoH 1994). With the correct individualized management and care, many people cope and recover from mental illness.

THE VALUE OF REFLEXOLOGY FOR PEOPLE WITH MENTAL HEALTH PROBLEMS

The relaxing effects of reflexology on people who are stressed, depressed, anxious or suffering from other mental health problems should not be underestimated (Sahai 1993, Shaw 1987, Trousdell 1996). The impact of touch on many of these people can be very profound (but care should be taken to identify those for whom touch is unwelcome). Although reflexology can never be a complete and discrete form of management of mental illness, it provides a pleasant, deeply relaxing and safe adjunct to conventional care, and frequently assists in relieving some of the physical effects associated with stress or depression (Box 13.1).

Box 13.1 Examples of physical or somatic symptoms associated with stress and/or depression (adapted from Donnellan 1997, Stuart & Sundeen 1995)

- Headaches
- Nausea
- Loss of appetite/overeating
- Weight loss/weight gain
- Bowel disturbance (diarrhoea or constipation)
- Muscle tension and pain
- Skin complaints, i.e. blotching, rashes, eczema
- Palpitations and sweating
- Breathing difficulties
- Tremor/shakiness
- Sleep disturbance
- Fatigue/exhaustion

The overall systemic relaxation effect of reflexology treatment can reduce headaches, heart rate and high systolic blood pressure (Dryden et al 1999, Frankel 1997, Lafuente et al 1997, Launso 1999), feelings of nausea or bowel disturbances such as diarrhoea or constipation (Eriksen 1995). Sleep should be more attainable and of better quality and musculoskeletal tensions may be relieved by working on the reflex zones specific to the areas of tension or pain. Alleviation of early gastrointestinal symptoms with reflexology may act in a preventive manner, so reducing the incidence of more serious problems such as duodenal ulcers. Boosting the immune system with regular reflexology treatment can contribute to a reduction in infections or skin complaints (Lett 2000).

The general impact of the treatment may assist in improving the client's self-esteem and reduce irritability, agitation and feelings of anger and loss of control. It has been reported that reflexology can help to improve mood and energy levels alongside creating a renewed or new-found interest in personal health and wellbeing (Mackereth, 1999, Trousdell 1996). This in turn may contribute to improving unhelpful coping strategies such as eating disorders, alcohol and substance abuse.

During a reflexology treatment the client has an opportunity for reflection on and non-judgemental discussion about his/her life. However, the practitioner should not give any advice which they are not qualified to give, nor attempt to impose their views or ideas but can facilitate the client to express fears or anxieties, explore options and empower them to make decisions for themselves. This can be a very effective approach in promoting autonomy and increased self-awareness and personal growth. Particular attention should be paid to the relevant reflex areas associated with stress such as the solar plexus, hypothalamus, pituitary and adrenal glands, as well as any other reflex points pertinent to physical symptoms being experienced (Kunz & Kunz 1993, Norman 1989).

Trust, respect, encouragement, communication and positive reinforcement all help the client to continue to make positive adjustments to lifestyle (Case study 13.1). The therapist needs to be aware of body language, such as facial expression and proximity, as this can communicate far more than speech, and in some cases it may not match verbal responses. For example, women may more readily admit to painful or tender reflex points during treatment than some male clients, who might judge admitting to pain as 'unmanly' or a failure. In order to be therapeutic, reflexology touch should be non-threatening and encourage relaxation, comfort and appropriate communication (Mackereth & Gale 1994). It is therefore important for the client to recognize the importance of disclosing any discomfort as this informs the treatment assessment and plan.

A welcoming therapeutic environment is necessary and will help to establish a trusting relationship between the client and the practitioner. Treatment may be provided in the home or a 'drop-in' centre or for those

---

Case study 13.1 Jan

Jan had suffered a phobia of confined spaces, was experiencing major difficulties in socializing with friends and was often having to make excuses to leave social situations. Her heart rate would rise, she would start to perspire and she would experience a shakiness and an overwhelming need to get out, all resulting in a sense of being out of control.

When Jan arrived for her first reflexology treatment her body language indicated that she was anxious and very uncomfortable. Jan and the reflexologist negotiated that if she felt a sense of panic and a need to leave the therapeutic space she could do so, without any explanation. This clearly gave her a sense of control, which she valued. Reflexology was performed regularly for several months and Jan felt that the sessions contributed greatly in reducing her levels of anxiety and gradually improving her ability to go out and socialize with friends.

Box 13.2 Reflexology contract issues for people with mental health problems

- Practitioners should establish whether a diagnosis of mental illness has already been made and identify any medication or therapy currently being administered.
- Liaison between the reflexologist and mental health workers who are already providing support, e.g. community psychiatric nurse, psychiatrist, counsellor or psychotherapist, is recommended (with consent from the client).
- Clients should be assessed to determine whether or not they are able to consent to and establish a therapeutic contract and that they understand fully the potential and limitations of treatment and the need to continue with conventional treatment (see also Box 13.3).
- Reflexologists must acknowledge their own parameters, prejudices and emotions and must take steps to ensure a comfortable working environment which is safe for both the practitioner and the client.

---

who are inpatients in a hospital setting, but privacy, confidentiality and adequate time are essential. A verbal or written therapeutic contract is one way of clarifying negotiations and setting boundaries (Box 13.2). Ongoing mutual evaluation assists in adapting and individualizing treatment in order to achieve its aims (Mackereth 1999).

CONCERNS, PRECAUTIONS AND CONTRAINDICATIONS TO REFLEXOLOGY

Reflexology, as with other complementary therapies can be helpful for people at times of crisis or transition (Cawthorn 2001) but it is important that the practitioner has a comprehensive knowledge of the individual's mental illness prior to offering treatment. One of the most valuable components of reflexology treatment for mental health clients is the time to talk over their problems, but it is essential that reflexologists who are not counsellors recognize their limitations and do not attempt to turn the session into a counselling event. If the practitioner also has responsibility for counselling of patients, as may be

> **Case study 13.2**   Ann
>
> On her third reflexology treatment, Ann, a married woman who supported her husband in the family business, mentioned how he generally ignored her and their conversations were always limited. Over the next few weeks Ann talked of her unhappiness and frustration. She was able to use the time while having reflexology to verbalize her feelings. She looked forward to the sessions because she was able to talk freely and become emotionally stronger. Later she arranged to see a counsellor with regard to her relationship problems.

the case for a nurse–reflexologist in a mental healthcare setting, it is important to differentiate times for reflexology and for counselling to take place.

It is important to acknowledge that touch is a powerful tool and patients may not inform the practitioner at the beginning of a therapeutic relationship that they have a past trauma such as sexual abuse or that they are in an unhappy relationship (Case study 13.2). Trust evolves in personal and professional relationships and these types of disclosure may not be revealed until weeks or months into reflexology treatment. To stay in role as a reflexologist and not to stray into counsellor mode can be difficult, particularly when a patient is obviously distressed or has shared their fears or past trauma with you. Being able to recognize the signs of the emergence of repressed feelings or the desire to unburden past or current hurt, worries or fears can be crucial in how we respond as reflexologists. Hoping that this will not happen or blocking emotional response by, for example, terminating the session or ignoring what has been said would be clearly unhelpful or even harmful. Preparatory education in becoming a reflexologist should include how to support an individual who becomes emotional or distressed.

Lett (2000) maintains that reflexologists in private practice should decline to treat people who are obviously experiencing extreme changes of mood, such as severe depression, manic states, paranoid ideas, or where there is an altered state of consciousness, as the impact of reflexology could potentially trigger a mental health crisis which the therapist will be ill-equipped to resolve. However, Mackereth (1999) in describing case studies where patients experienced strong emotional responses to treatment, states that reflexologists do have a role to play. This can include supporting the patient in seeking counselling support and having the interpersonal skills to be with the person as they express their distress.

WORKING WITH PEOPLE WHO HAVE ACUTE AND/OR ENDURING MENTAL HEALTH PROBLEMS

Importantly, this area of practice requires the reflexologist to have experience in mental health care and knowledge of mental illness and statutory provision. Clinical support and supervision for their work should be in place, preferably with a supervisor who has expertise and skills in the field of mental health. Typically, supervision is an activity that involves a contracted and formal arrangement with a supervisor to review and reflect upon clinical work to enable the further development of professional practice (Faugier & Butterworth 1994). Most commonly this involves meeting either as a member of a supervision group or a one-to-one arrangement (see Chapter 2). Models of supervision within the mental health professions, such as nursing, counselling and psychotherapy, have a long history and can be adapted for use with complementary therapists (Mackereth 2001).

People being treated by conventional means should receive reflexology only after consultation with the medical team. If there are any doubts or apprehensions about treating people who are mentally ill, reflexology should be withheld and the client should be advised to contact the GP. Clients who insist on receiving reflexology should be referred to a practitioner with more specific expertise.

Reflexologists should work only within the boundaries of their own knowledge and experience of people with mental health needs. A client experiencing extreme levels of anxiety and stress may be unpredictable and pose a danger to themselves and others, including the reflexologist, for example by hitting out, throwing objects or self-harm (Newell & Gournay 2000). An initial assessment of the client, perhaps by telephone, should attempt to determine how anxiety or stress affects behaviour and whether or not reflexology would be appropriate. With all client groups, safety must be a primary consideration. Practitioners working in a clinical area with patients who have challenging behaviour must be aware of policies and practices to best assess and manage these situations. It is not always easy, even for an experienced psychiatric nurse, to predict a person's behaviour and incidents may occur for which patients need specialist help and support in times of crisis. Again, supervision is a means of ongoing support for those electing to work in this challenging area of practice.

ETHICAL AND LEGAL CONCERNS

All reflexology practitioners need to have an awareness of the ethical and legal principles of informed consent, as this is a crucial issue in clinical practice. Practitioners need to be aware of any special needs within their client group that may have an influence on giving informed consent, such as persons receiving treatment under the Mental Health Act (DoH 1983) and mentally incapacitated adults. The Mental Health Act (currently under review) governs legislation for consent to psychiatric treatment (DoH 1999). It is important, however, that the reflexologist does not assume that persons receiving care under the Mental Health Act are not competent to give informed consent. The practitioner should work on the premise that clients are competent to consent (UKCC 1998). However, care needs to be exercised to ensure the client can understand and retain information and has the ability to appraise information given (Dunn 1998). Some clients may have a fluctuating state of competence and it is necessary for the reflexologist to assess that these clients continue to understand and give their consent. There should also be awareness by the practitioner that compliance does not necessarily mean consent (UKCC 1998). The word 'consent' comes from the Latin *consentire*, which means to feel or think together. For consent to be valid and informed, the client needs to understand the nature and consequences of the proposed treatment. The practitioner needs to communicate this information and be reassured that the client comprehends the proposed intervention. There are a variety of definitions and theories of reflexology (Chapter 1), so it requires the practitioner to assess carefully what language to use that best facilitates an informed choice. A patient's anxiety can also hamper communication, so any discussion about consent must not be hurried or pressured. Providing information ahead of making a decision, possibly even by days or weeks, may provide the patient with the time to reflect on whether they really do wish to participate in reflexology.

Clinical policies and guidelines on consent must be adhered to and, additionally, reflexologists will also need to be guided by their governing body's Code of Professional Conduct. Verbal or written consent is accepted by law, however, evidence of consent is advisable (Dimond 1998) and, in the area of mental health and learning disability, accurate recording of communications leading to consent is recommended (UKCC 1998). Practitioners working within the NHS and other healthcare services require consent from their employer and the doctor clinically responsible for the client's care (Dimond 1998). Recommendation for best practice in eliciting and maintaining informed consent for reflexology is detailed in Box 13.3.

SUMMARY: A MODEL OF REFLEXOLOGY PRACTICE IN MENTAL HEALTH

- Attending to the whole person is essential if reflexology is to be a positive and helpful intervention.
- Touch can be very powerful and care must be taken to best manage cathartic responses to treatment.
- Reflexologists need to stay in role but be able to support patients in an appropriate and helpful manner, for example, by referral to mental health practitioners prior to treatment.
- Reflexologists must ensure that best practice is adopted with regard to eliciting and maintaining informed consent (see Box 13.3).

Box 13.3   Eliciting and maintaining informed consent for reflexology

- If the referral is from another healthcare worker the request will need to have been discussed and agreed with the patient.
- Ensure that when beginning the consent process the patient is able to communicate with you and that their judgement is not compromised by the severity of the illness, medication (prescribed and non-prescribed) or alcohol.
- Explain the intended reflexology intervention, including the possible benefits to the client, contraindications and potential side-effects.
- Check that the client has understood and is satisfied with the information you have given.
- Provide written information and encourage the client to take time to reflect on all information given and options available before decision taken. This might include discussion with the mental healthcare worker, advocate, family and friends.
- Gain agreement/consent (preferably written) to the proposed course of reflexology treatment (Dimond 1995).
- Explain that the client can withdraw consent at any stage of treatment. This could include the patient testing the 'stop' to touch in the first session, so affirming the patient's right to say 'no' to touch at any point in bodywork practices (Mackereth 2000).
- Review the treatment with the client from time to time, to confirm ongoing understanding and consent.

- Safety and protection are crucial for both the practitioner and patient. For example, it would be inappropriate for reflexologists to treat patients who are psychotic or under the influence of alcohol or illicit drugs.
- Obtain clinical supervision for your work, ideally from a supervisor with experience in mental health and complementary therapies.

CONCLUSION

Clients come for reflexology for all sorts of reasons, and may continue treatments because they are pleasantly surprised that they can be empowered at the same time. As Mackereth suggests, being listened to by a skilled practitioner 'whose focus is your well-being through physical nurturing contact' (Mackereth 1999 p 69) may be a new and enriching experience for some individuals. It is not uncommon to find that many clients with mental health problems want that experience of being nurtured and supported. Empowerment can be facilitated with the support of reflexology practitioners who are able to be compassionate, present and focused in their work with clients. Being positive and encouraging as a therapist can help to promote positive thinking for the client. That can only come about if the practitioner is confident, knowledgeable about mental health issues and supported in their work. Naidoo & Wills (1994 p 89) describe empowerment as an approach that 'enables people to identify their own concerns and gain the skills and confidence to act upon them'. As a package, reflexology can encompass emotional, spiritual and physical support and healing.

However, to be truly powerful as a treatment it also requires both the practitioner and client to be committed and engage in the work.

Not everyone who has mental health needs will have access to reflexology through the NHS, but times are changing and the availability of complementary therapies within the NHS is increasing. Orthodox medicine and treatment is vital in helping people recover from mental ill health, but healthcare professionals are clearly increasingly recognizing that complementary therapies can be integrated with positive results (Archer 1999). Reflexology, when delivered by skilled practitioners, with awareness and knowledge of mental health issues, can expand the treatment options for people affected by mental health problems.

REFERENCES

Archer C. Research issues in complementary therapies. Complementary Therapies in Nursing and Midwifery 1999; 5:108–114.
Boseley S. Are we really more miserable? Guardian Unlimited. Online. Available: http://www.guardian.co.uk 16 May 2001.
Cawthorn A. Communication skills and counselling. In: Rankin-Box D, ed. The nurse's handbook of complementary therapies. Edinburgh: Ballière Tindall; 2001.
Department of Health (DoH). Mental Health Act (1983). London: HMSO; 1983.
Department of Health (DoH). Working in partnership: a collaborative approach to care. Report of the Mental Health Nursing Review Team. London: Department of Health/HMSO; 1994.
Department of Health (DoH). Reform of the Mental Health Act 1983 – a green paper. London: Department of Health/HMSO; 1999.
Dimond B. The legal aspects of complementary therapy practice. Edinburgh: Churchill Livingstone; 1998.
Donnellan C. Mental illness, vol. 21. Milton Keynes: City Print Ltd; 1997.
Dryden SL, Holden SD, Mackereth P. "Just the ticket": the findings of a pilot complementary service (Part II). Complementary Therapies in Nursing and Midwifery 1999; 5:15–18.
Dunn C. Ethical issues in mental illness. Aldershot: Ashgate Publishers; 1998.
Eriksen L. Using reflexology to relieve chronic constipation. In: Danish Reflexologists Association: a collection of articles. Denmark: Danish Reflexologists' Association; 1995.
Faugier J, Butterworth T. Clinical supervision: a position paper. Manchester: School of Nursing Studies, University of Manchester; 1994.
Frankel B. The effect of reflexology on barreceptor reflex sensitivity, blood pressure and sinus arrhythmia. Complementary Therapies in Medicine 1997; 5:80–84.
Holmes TH, Rahe RH. The social readjustment rating scale. Journal of Psychosomatic Research 1967; 11:213–218.
Kunz K, Kunz B. The complete guide to foot reflexology. Albuquerque, NM: Reflexology Research; 1993.
Lafuente A, Nouera M, Puy C, et al. Effects of treatment with stimulation of the reflex zones of the foot with regard to the prophylactic Flunarizin™ treatment of patients suffering from headaches (first published 1990). Reprinted in Reflexology Research Reports. 4th edn. London: Association of Reflexologists; 1997: 39–40.
Launso L, Brendstrup E, Arnberg S. An exploratory study of reflexological treatment for headache. Alternative Therapies 1999; 5(3):57–65.
Lett A. Reflex zone therapy for health professionals. Edinburgh: Churchill Livingstone; 2000.
Mackereth PA. Tough places to be tender: contracting for happy or 'good enough' endings in therapeutic massage/bodywork? Complementary Therapies in Nursing and Midwifery 2000; 6(3):111–115.

Mackereth PA. An introduction to catharsis and the healing crisis in reflexology. Complementary Therapies in Nursing and Midwifery 1999; 5:67–74.

Mackereth PA. Clinical supervision. In: Rankin-Box D, ed. The nurse's handbook of complementary therapies. 2nd edn. Edinburgh: Ballière Tindall; 2001.

Mackereth PA, Gale E. Touch/massage workshops – a pilot study. Complementary Therapies in Medicine 1994; 2:93–98.

Naidoo J, Wills J. Health promotion. Foundations for practice. London: Baillière Tindall; 1994.

Newell R, Gournay K. Mental health nursing: an evidence-based approach. London: Churchill Livingstone; 2000.

Norman L. The reflexology handbook. London: Piatkus; 1989.

Sahai CM. Reflexology – its place in modern healthcare. Professional Nurse 1993; 8(11): 722–725.

Shaw J. Reflexology. Health Visitor 1987; 60(11):367.

Stuart GW, Sundeen SJ. Principles of psychiatric nursing. 5th edn. St Louis: CV Mosby; 1995.

Trousdell P. Reflexology meets emotional needs. International Journal of Alternative and Complementary Medicine 1996; November: 9–12.

UKCC. Guidelines for mental health and learning disabilities. London: United Kingdom Central Council for Nursing, Midwifery and Health Visiting; 1998.

USEFUL ADDRESSES

MIND (The National Association for Mental Health)
Granta House, 15–19 Broadway, London, E15 4BQ
Tel: 0208 519 2122
Information line: 0845 766 0163

A mental health charity which aims to raise public awareness of mental health issues and works for the rights of mentally ill people to lead an active and valued life in the community.

The Samaritans
10 The Grove, Slough, SL1 1QP
Tel: 01753 532713
Helpline: 0345 909090

Exists to provide confidential, emotional support at any hour of the day or night to those people passing through emotional crisis and in danger of taking their own lives.

SANE
First Floor,
Cityside House,
40 Alder Street, London, E1 1EE
Tel: 0207 375 1002
SANELINE: 0845 767 8000

SANE's national telephone helpline, SANELINE, offers support and a range of practical information to anyone coping with mental illness, and their carers, relatives or friends.

Triumph Over Phobia (TOP UK)
PO Box 1831, Bath, BA1 3YX
Tel: 01225 330353

Provides help, support and advice to people with phobias, obsessive compulsive disorder and associated panics.

14

Enhancing quality of life for people in palliative care settings

Edwina Hodkinson and Julia M. Williams

Supporting people with a life-limiting
  condition
  Physical support
  Emotional support
  Spiritual support
Dispelling the myths
Adapting reflexology in palliative care

Working with carers
Conclusion
References
Further reading
Useful addresses
Acknowledgements

Abstract

Reflexology can be a very positive experience for patients and their carers in palliative care and haemato-oncology settings. This chapter aims to examine fears and myths about working with people who have cancer and other life-limiting illnesses and to suggest ways of adapting reflexology to meet specific needs and manage certain symptoms. Most importantly, the chapter debates key issues surrounding the integration of clinical reflexology into conventional care for people in palliative care settings.

  The chapter does not address the issue of reflexologists in independent practice who may see people with cancer or chronic progressive illness in their private clinics. However, it should be noted that, under the Cancer Act 1939, it is illegal to take sole responsibility for the treatment of people with cancer or to make any guarantee or promise of 'cure' with reflexology.

Key words: palliation, myths, hope, treatment adaptation, inclusion

A staggering 40% of people will be affected by cancer at some time in their life, and for many the care will be palliative rather than curative (Daniel 2001 p 9). Palliative care has been described as the full and 'active' care of patients and their families by a multi-professional team at a time when the disease has become unresponsive to 'curative' treatment (WHO 1990). Increasingly, others will face the frightening and distressing experience of the diagnosis and prognosis of a life-threatening disease, such as auto-immune deficiency syndrome (AIDS), cardiovascular disease, chronic lung disease or multiple sclerosis. As well as the associated symptoms of the disease there will be the iatrogenic effects from treatments, often worse than the disease. Treatments impact on the body, self-image and confidence, especially disfiguring surgery or cytotoxic chemotherapy that leads to hair loss, or high-dose steroids that cause significant changes in weight. The impact on finances, work, family life and personal relationships can be significant; those affected can feel lonely, isolated and afraid.

The World Health Organization (1990) identified the goals of palliative care as assisting patients and their families to achieve the best possible quality of life in the time that is left, including control of pain and other symptoms and management of other aspects of their lives. Complementary therapies, including reflexology, offer a holistic approach which provides physical, emotional and spiritual support (Kohn 1999). An estimated one-third of cancer patients use complementary therapies regularly as an adjunct to conventional treatment (Kohn 1999) and 70% of cancer/palliative care units now provide a range of complementary therapies (Centrepiece 2000), with touch therapies, including reflexology, the most widely used (Byass 1999, Penson 1998). Reflexology can make a valuable contribution to health care by providing support and enhancing quality of life for patients and their families, as well as having therapeutic benefits in terms of symptom relief (Kassab & Stevensen 1996).

SUPPORTING PEOPLE WITH A LIFE-LIMITING CONDITION

PHYSICAL SUPPORT

Reflexology can be a valuable supportive treatment in the alleviation of many physical problems and side-effects of treatment, particularly in the relief of pain through the production of endorphins from its relaxation effects (Grealish et al 2000, Stephenson & Weinrich 2000). Reflexology may help with physical symptoms caused by chemotherapy or radiotherapy, such as constipation, diarrhoea and nausea (Grealish et al 2000, Hodgeson 2000, Hodkinson 2001). Reflexology and other forms of soft tissue massage may boost the immune system (McNamara 1993), assisting those with compromised immunity associated with chemotherapy or radiotherapy to resist infection. It has also been suggested that working reflex areas not only relaxes the body but can also 'conserve' energy levels (Bechterev 1932/ 1973).

EMOTIONAL SUPPORT

Reflexology is a powerful and significant form of non-verbal communication, which fulfils the basic human need to be touched. Ill people are sometimes touched only in a very mechanical way, either in the provision of basic care or during uncomfortable procedures, whereas touch during a reflexology treatment can be positive and therapeutic, offering comfort, warmth and friendship without being intimidating in any way. For a person who is dying, this form of touch can be very soothing and helps the person to realize that the body can still provide pleasure as well as pain. The deep relaxation achieved by reflexology helps to relieve mental stress, aid sleep and rest, and provides a coping mechanism for depression and anxiety (Trousdell 1996) through the release of suppressed emotion (Mackereth 1999). This can empower people to develop a more positive approach to the situation and to feel more able to cope with their illness and treatment, as well as to enjoy a better quality of life (Hodgeson 2000, Stephenson & Weinrich 2000)

SPIRITUAL SUPPORT

People with a life-limiting illness often undertake a purposeful search for meaning, forgiveness, hope and love (Elsdon 1995), perhaps making an inward journey, questioning sometimes long-held beliefs and ideals. Elsdon (1995) believes that supporting this spiritual work is vital for a patient's wellbeing and that if those needs are met there will usually be significantly lower levels of anxiety. Kubler Ross (1969) has identified a number of psychological stages in the process of coming to terms with impending death, and the support of carers can be invaluable in facilitating patients to find inner strength, spiritual growth and peace (Mitchell & Cormack 1998). The nature of a reflexology treatment provides patients with the undivided, face-to-face attention of the therapist with time and opportunity to talk about their innermost feelings and fears (Hodkinson 2001) when they may otherwise be unable to express themselves in this way for fear of upsetting family and friends (Bristol Oncology Centre et al 1999). This requires the practitioner to be sufficiently experienced and knowledgeable to deal with the situation sensitively and appropriately, and also requires the therapist to find a time to debrief for his or her own wellbeing (Cassidy 1998).

DISPELLING THE MYTHS

Practitioners intending to provide reflexology for people with cancer may encounter controversial and differing opinions as many quote cancer, radiotherapy and chemotherapy as contraindications to receiving reflexology (see Chapter 3), perhaps in an attempt to protect patients from novice or inexperienced practitioners. Reflexologists should be experienced, understand fully the diseases and their treatments, work in conjunction with consultants and other team members and be able to adapt treatments appropriately in order to avoid adverse reactions.

Concerns have been raised about reflexology overstimulating lymphatic and circulatory flow, thus allowing cancer cells to metastasize (Kassab & Stevensen 1996, McNamara 1993), although oncologists now believe that intended metastases will occur irrespective of whether the patient receives massage or reflexology, and some, such as Professor Sikora at Hammersmith Hospital in London, are vociferous in their support of the use of massage and reflexology, provided skilled practitioners deliver them as gentle and complementary adjuncts to conventional care (Bell & Sikora 1996). Kassab & Stevensen (1996) suggest that blood circulation and lymphatic flow can be stimulated by everyday activities such as having a hot bath, or walking upstairs, as much, if not more, than by the gentle actions of reflexology, and that this concern is misguided through lack of pathology and physiological knowledge.

Chemotherapy is found by patients to be an extremely tiring, very depressing and unpleasant experience (Izod 1996). It has been suggested that reflexology might interfere with the effects of chemotherapeutic drugs (Kassab & Stevensen 1996), although these authors have found no evidence to support or refute this belief. Indeed, anecdotal reports suggest that reflexology provides relief from the associated nausea, vomiting and constipation that is common during chemotherapy (Grealish et al 2000, Hodkinson 2001, Stephenson & Weinrich 2000) and aids restful sleep following treatment (Izod 1996) (see Case study 14.1). It is thought that touch therapies such as reflexology can limit the effects of stress on normal cells of the body, so strengthening the body as a whole (Kassab & Stevensen 1996) and supporting the immune system depleted during chemotherapy. However, the medium- to short-term side-effects of chemotherapy and high-dose steroids need to be considered, for example, loss of skin integrity and thrombocytopenia, both contributing to poor skin healing and bruising. It is therefore essential to examine the condition of the patient's skin carefully and note any bruising or tendency to bleed easily before embarking upon treatment.

Case study 14.1 Ann

Ann, a 46-year-old woman with pancreatic cancer and localized spread to her liver, stomach, bowel, spleen and kidney had coped well with extensive abdominal surgery and had just commenced a second course of chemotherapy, about which she was very anxious as she had experienced severe vomiting during the first course. She was referred by her GP for reflexology as a means of helping her to relax and cope with the impact of her illness and the treatment.

Reflexology was given from the day before the chemotherapy and Ann noticed the difference immediately. Normally she experienced severe nausea for 2 days following chemotherapy but this did not occur at all. She felt very relaxed, less fatigued and was able to sleep better. No morphine was required for breakthrough pain and no consequent constipation ensued.

Radiotherapy is also a stressful and tiring experience, especially for out-patients travelling to hospital from home and then waiting anxiously to receive their treatment. Fatigue appears to increase as the treatment progresses, perhaps partly due to the underlying disease process and partly to the radiotherapy side-effects, including nausea, vomiting, anaemia and bone marrow depression (Spreadborough & Read 2000). There is, however, no theoretical basis for reflexology interfering with the effects of the radiotherapy; rather, it can offer relaxation and promote recuperation, particularly if given regularly during the treatment. Dry skin can be a problem for people undergoing radiotherapy; this may be localized to the area of treatment or more generalized. Some radiologists will not permit direct tissue pressure to areas actually being treated (Horrigan 2001). Reflexologists need to be thoroughly familiar with the patient's particular radiotherapy treatment and take into account the skin prior to commencing the session.

There are very few contraindications to performing reflexology for people with cancer but care must focus on informed consent, safety and comfort. The most fundamental contraindication would be if the patient declines treatment or if relatives will not consent to the therapist working with a patient who is unable to make that choice. Practitioners who have or think they may be suffering from contagious infections such as a cold, influenza, diarrhoea, vomiting, or who are feeling unwell should not be in contact with patients whose immune system is compromised by the effects of cytotoxic chemotherapy, radiotherapy, high-dose steroids, blood/marrow transplantation or disease involvement of the bone marrow such as leukaemia. Patients with haemato-oncological disease will experience a period of pancytopenia predisposing them to neutropenia, thrombocytopenia and anaemia. It is therefore essential to adapt reflexology treatment and to work very gently and with caution over the skin.

ADAPTING REFLEXOLOGY IN PALLIATIVE CARE

Reflexology treatment can be given almost anywhere, from a specially equipped therapy room to the patient's living room or bedroom (Hodkinson 2001), or even the garden on a summer's day. People can receive reflexology in a chair, wheelchair or bed. In hospital or a hospice, treatment can be given at the bedside of a very sick person or someone close to death, providing relaxation and comfort. Access to reflexology services in hospitals or hospices can be very welcoming for newly admitted patients who will be feeling vulnerable, frightened and lonely. If the person is being cared for at home, teamwork with other healthcare professionals such as Macmillan and Marie Curie nurses, social workers and GPs can never be underestimated and may require the reflexologist to coordinate timing of sessions with other elements of the person's care.

The person's health may vary enormously from day to day and the feet and hands may vary in sensitivity. The perception of touch and pressure may be affected by chronic illness or medication such as strong analgesics, steroids, hypnotics, tranquillizers and narcotics. Tumours of the central nervous system can deeply alter peripheral sensation, for example, spinal tumours causing cord compression may result in numbness of the whole or part of the foot or feet. Sensory perception may also be influenced by the person's psychological state. Neuropathy of the feet and hands can be a chronic or worsening symptom of diseases such as multiple sclerosis and the reflexologist must be able to assess the condition of the reflexes and adapt treatment accordingly so that the feet are not overstimulated in any way. Patients with neuropathy may benefit from a long course of reflexology and psychological and spiritual aspects of treatment may be more important than physical effects. Extremely light touch may be necessary on some occasions whilst on others a deeper treatment will help to ease symptoms. Different techniques may also be necessary, such as incorporating lymphatic drainage into the basic treatment if the patient has developed ankle oedema due to immobility. However, not all patients will have altered sensation in the feet and hands and some will present with normal reflexes and sensations. For these patients, pressures are adapted according to the discretion of the therapist and the preferences of the patient.

The frequency and duration of reflexology treatments must be individualized and caution should be exercised during the first session to avoid strong reactions. Treatment duration may be as short as 20 minutes or up to 50 minutes, depending upon the patient's health, reaction to the session and the reason for undertaking it, but shorter, more frequent treatments may suit some patients. Reflexology can be a very potent therapy and quality of treatment is more important than quantity when dealing with the very sick. To adapt and be flexible is the key to a rewarding experience for both the client and the practitioner.

Practitioners must be considerate of themselves in this work – emotionally, physically and spiritually. Care must be taken with posture when working with patients confined to bed or in a wheelchair. Physically, working at an awkward angle can cause discomfort, pain, injury or repetitive strain (see Chapter 8). This type of work can be emotionally distressing and unresolved bereavement issues should be addressed through supervision, mentoring and debriefing. Care must be taken to ensure that the patient does not unintentionally become a distraction or that the therapist does not continually relive failure, guilt or sadness of previous losses. An unconditional, professional yet caring approach as a therapist requires conscious reflection, so that we can be present for others and identify when we need support and supervision (see Chapter 2).

Ideally, reflexology should be applied to the whole foot at every treatment, especially with people with systemic conditions such as leukaemia.

Gentle and sensitive palpation should be performed over the zones relating to the location of tumours but patients often report that attention to these zones relieves pain in the tumour location. If the tumour is located on the spinal cord, reflexology appears to dispel congestion and facilitate an increased awareness of the lower body from which the person might have felt disconnected (Case study 14.2). After surgery, awareness of the tumour location is equally important to aid recovery and recuperation.

People with HIV and AIDS may develop a range of complications, including Karposi's sarcoma, a cancer that can be present on the lower legs and feet, and fungal and viral-related pedal skin conditions, and care should be taken to avoid working directly on the affected area. It has been noted by these authors and others that the patches of Karposi's sarcoma appear to occur on areas of the feet that relate to the patient's internal problems. If the person is suffering neuropathy, a severe sensitivity or numbness of the legs and feet, pressure must be applied very sensitively or the therapist may opt to work on the patient's hands (Fig. 14.1, Plate 17). Reflexology can also be useful in reducing stress levels to enhance the immune function and to assist the person in tolerating the side-effects of drugs.

Elderly people are most often in need of touch and yet are the least likely to receive it (Montague 1986), and reflexology can be a very practical yet caring treatment which they will enjoy, not least because treatment on the feet is less intrusive than other manual therapies such as massage of the back. The older person's feet often present a challenge in terms of their mobility and circulatory problems, but the touch of reflexology can often visibly soften the expression on the client's face while the muscles of the whole body seem to relax.

Case study 14.2   Angela

Angela's diagnosis of leukaemia was a tremendous shock to her husband, a doctor, and her two children. Angela requested reflexology and when she had her first session shortly after starting a course of chemotherapy she expressed a feeling of disconnectedness in 'body and spirit'. Gentle reflexology was used with the aim of 'bringing her together' again. Stroking the foot zones for the spine elicited a 'tingling through the body, like electricity' which seemed to help Angela to feel whole again.

Later, Angela was admitted to the intensive care unit needing artificial ventilation and, despite his earlier scepticism, her husband recognized the benefits of the previous reflexology and requested that she receive it again. Angela had three sessions during her week in the intensive care unit and both clinical and emotional effects were observed after each treatment. Angela's condition stabilized and she returned to the ward where some weeks later she died peacefully.

Her husband later came back to the unit to receive reflexology because it had meant so much to his wife. He felt it would help him to cope with his grief and increase his stamina to look after his young family.

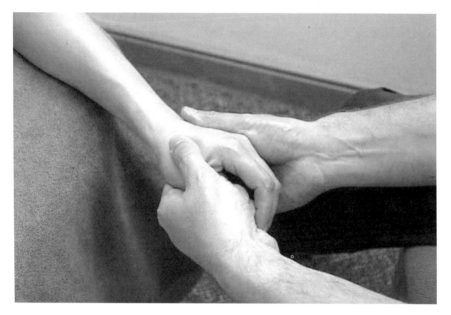

Figure 14.1 Practitioner working at the bedside on the hand (see also Plate 17). Photo courtesy of Katie Spruce BA (Hons), medical photographer, Christie Hospital NHS Trust, with permission.

WORKING WITH CARERS

A diagnosis of terminal illness is frightening and stressful not only for the patient but also for the whole family, close friends and those who are caring for the person. It has a profound impact on personal relationships (Bristol Oncology Centre et al 1999). A desire to protect the patient from the full impact of the disease, 'putting on a brave face' and attempting to provide daily care is physically and emotionally draining and carers may sometimes be neglectful of themselves. They may also have the pressure of coping with young families, jobs and financial concerns. It is in these situations that reflexology can have enormous benefit. Many people with cancer also worry about their loved ones and the knowledge that they are receiving beneficial treatment can be very reassuring.

Reflexology may help relatives and carers to take time out and focus on their own needs, providing an opportunity to talk to a professional not directly involved in the situation, which can frequently evoke a cathartic release. Relief of existing physical problems and ailments can give relatives extra strength to carry on and can act as a preventative measure against illness and infections, which may result from a stressed immune system (MacDonald 1999). If they are able to continue with treatment after the death of their loved one, then reflexology can be of help in the grieving process in a positive way (Case study 14.3).

Case study 14.3   Susan

Susan's mother was in the terminal stages of lung cancer and Susan was caring for her at home whilst also trying to continue working. On the surface she seemed calm and appeared to be coping well but she agreed to receive reflexology as a 'treat' for herself. The areas on her feet corresponding to the solar plexus, adrenal glands and neck were very tender. As Susan relaxed she started to talk about her mother and about death. Towards the end of the treatment her hands perspired profusely, she started to giggle and commented on how 'high' she felt – 'like being on drugs'. Susan cancelled the next treatment but her brother contacted the reflexologist to report that, after the treatment, not only did her neck, back and shoulders ache but she cried, shouted, was angry and felt 'completely out of control' with her emotions. This emotional release frightened Susan, but her brother commented on how relieved the whole family was that this had happened, as they had been so worried about her.

CONCLUSION

Dispelling myths and worries about using reflexology in palliative care settings is about educating practitioners, potential users and providers of complementary therapy services, multi-professional team members and teachers of reflexology/CAM. It is also important for others working in cancer/palliative care settings to audit, evaluate through research and share their expertise and understanding with the wider public and health professionals.

When reflexology is provided in a palliative care setting it is essential that the patient is at the centre of the treatment process because living and dying is ultimately a unique, intimate and personal journey. Reflexology can offer a means of relieving physical symptoms and of facilitating emotional and spiritual wellbeing, but requires the therapist to practise with awareness, sensitivity, intuition and adaptability. Reflexology cannot promise sustained improvements in physical health but can provide therapeutic touch and the space and attention to support patients in connecting their mind, body and spirit.

Reflexology can also be invaluable in helping carers to cope both before and after the death of their loved ones. It is vital that reflexologists acknowledge their contribution within the team of professionals involved in caring for the person and the family and the need for practice to be based on contemporary evidence-based knowledge. Sensitivity and humility enable the practitioner to provide holistic, individualized and appropriate care for people at perhaps the most difficult time of their lives.

REFERENCES

Bechterev VM. General Principles of Reflexology. First printed 1932, reprinted (and translated from Russian) 1973, New York: Arno Press, Inc.

Bell L, Sikora K. Complementary therapies and cancer care. Complementary Therapies in Nursing and Midwifery 1996; 2(3):57–58.

Bristol Oncology Centre, University of Warwick, Bristol Cancer Help Centre. Meeting the needs of people with cancer for support and self-management – a collaborative report. Bristol: Bristol Cancer Help Centre; 1999.

Byass R. Auditing complementary therapies in palliative care: the experience of the day-care massage service at Mount Edgcumbe Hospice. Complementary Therapies in Nursing and Midwifery 1999; 5(2):51–60.

Cassidy S. Sharing the darkness, the spirituality of caring. London: Darton, Longman and Todd; 1988.

CentrePiece. The newsletter of the Bristol Cancer Help Centre. Spring 2000; issue 34:1.

Daniel R. The cancer prevention book. London: Simon and Schuster; 2001.

Davies P. The power of Touch. Carlsbad, California: Hay House Inc; 1999.

Elsdon R. Spiritual pain in dying people: the nurse's role. Professional Nurse 1995; 10(10):641–643.

Grealish L, Lomasney A, Whiteman B. Foot massage: a nursing intervention to modify the distressing symptoms of pain and nausea in patients hospitalised with cancer. Cancer Nursing 2000. 23(3):237–243.

Hodgeson H. Does reflexology impact on cancer patient's quality of life? Nursing Standard 2000. 14(31):33–38.

Hodkinson E. The benefits of reflexology in palliative care. Reflexions The Journal of the Association of Reflexologists 2001; issue 63:27.

Horrigan C. Massage. In: Rankin-Box D, ed. The nurse's handbook of complementary therapies. 2nd edn. London: Harcourt Publishers; 2001.

Izod D. A patient's perspective. Complementary Therapies in Nursing and Midwifery 1996; 2(3):66–67.

Kassab S, Stevensen C. Common misunderstandings about complementary therapies for people with cancer. Complementary Therapies in Nursing and Midwifery 1996; 2(3):62–65.

Kohn M. Complementary therapies in cancer care. London: Macmillan Cancer Relief; 1999.

Kubler Ross E. On death and dying. New York: TouchStone; 1969.

MacDonald G. Medicine hands, massage therapy for people with cancer. Tallahassee, Florida: 1999.

Mackereth PA. An introduction to catharsis and the healing crisis in reflexology. Complementary Therapies in Nursing and Midwifery 1999; 5(3):67–74.

McNamara P. Massage for people with cancer. London: Wandsworth Cancer Support Centre; 1993.

Mitchell A, Cormack M. The therapeutic relationship in complementary health care. London: Churchill Livingstone; 1998.

Montague A. Touching, the human significance of the skin. 3rd edn. New York: Harper and Row Publishers; 1986.

Penson J. Complementary therapies: making a difference in palliative care. Complementary Therapies in Nursing and Midwifery 1998; 4(3):77–81.

Spreadborough D, Read J. Radiotherapy. In: Grundy E, ed. Nursing in Haematological Oncology. London: Harcourt Publishers; 2000.

Stephenson NLN, Weinrich SP. The effects of foot reflexology on anxiety and pain in patients with breast and lung cancer. Oncology Nursing Forum 2000; 27(1):67–72.

Trousdell P. Reflexology meets emotional needs. International Journal of Alternative and Complementary Medicine 1996; November: 9–12.

World Health Organization (WHO). Cancer pain relief and palliative care. Report of WHO Expert Committee. Technical Report Series no. 804. Geneva: WHO; 1990.

FURTHER READING

Callanan M, Kelley P. Final Gifts. London: Bantam; 1997.

De Hennezel M. Intimate death (trans. C. Janeway). London: Warner Books; 1997.

Levine S. Meetings at the edge. Bath: Gateway Books; 1984 (reprinted 1996).
Rinpoche S. Tibetan Book of Living and Dying. London: Rider; 1993.

USEFUL ADDRESSES

National Association of Complementary Therapists in Hospice and Palliative Care
32 Milner Road, Selly Park, Birmingham, B29 7RQ
Tel: 0121 472 4987

Teenage Cancer Trust
Kirkman House, Kirkman Place, 54a Tottenham Court Road, London, W1P 9RF
Tel: 0207 436 2877
Fax: 0207 637 4302
E-mail:tct@teencancer.bdx.co.uk
Website: http://www.teencancer.org

Macmillan Cancer Relief Macmillan Fund
15–19 Britten Street, London, SW3 TZ
Tel: 0207 352 7811

CancerBacup
3 Bath Place, Rivington Street, London, EC2A 3JR
Tel: 0207 613 2121

Marie Curie Cancer Care
28 Belgrave Square, London, SW1X 8QG
Tel: 0207 235 3325

Bristol Cancer Help Centre
Grove House, Cornwallis Grove, Clifton, Bristol, BS8 4PG
Tel: 01272 743216

ACKNOWLEDGEMENTS

With thanks to Timothy Jackson, Divisional Nurse Director of Nursing Services, Royal Marsden Hospital, London, for help with preparing this chapter.

Index

Essential oils, using
learning disabled people, 164
in pregnancy, 136, 141
Ethical issues, 53
duty to benefit and not harm, 54–57
mental health clients, 176–177
respecting autonomy, 58
Evaluation, treatment, 100
Examination of feet, 13–14
'Expressive' touch, 160, 161

F

Falling, 'No Hands' reflexology, 109
Fatigue, treatment-induced, 10
'Feet as the U bend theory', 12
Feng Shui, 86
Fitzgerald, William, 6, 9
Flow, 'No Hands' reflexology, 109
Foot charts, 6, 7–8, 40–43, **49–50**
'Foot mangle' technique, 110–111, **112**
Forearm, use of, 'No Hands' approach,
110–111, **112**, **114**
Foundation for Integrated Medicine (FIM),
24–25, 33, 127
research questions and methodology, **62**
Frankel study, physiological effects,
reflexology, 9, 66–67, 73
'Functional' touch, 160, 161
Funding, hospital reflexology, 126, 129

G

Gate control theory, 9
General health, improving, 162
General practitioners (GPs), 37
General Reflexology Council (GRC), 26
Gillanders, Ann, 19
'Grounding', 109

H

Haemorrhage, postpartum, 144
Hand reflexology, **188**
breast points, 155
chart, **51**
in lower limb impairment, 162
Hara, 109
Headache
management in pregnancy, 139, 140
mothers in neonatal unit, 154
research trials, 64–65, 73, 74
Healing, 79–82
environments for, 85–86
healing crisis, 80–82, 99

see also Catharsis
and holism, 78–79
see also Spirituality
Health and Beauty departments, 20–21
see also 'Salon reflexology'
Healthcare Trusts, 122, 123
Healthwork UK, 25
Higher education institutions, 22–24
Historical perspectives, 5–7
HIV, 187
Holism, healing and, 78–79
Holistic frameworks for care, 95–96
Holistic Healing Centre, 19
Holistic multidimensional system, 7
Home remedy, constipation relief, 141
Hospice movement, 85
see also Palliative care settings
Hospitalization, stress of, 122
Hume's behaviour therapy model, 96
Hyperemesis gravidarum, 139
case study, 140
Hyperthyroidism, 172
Hypothalamus reflex zone, 39, 40, **41**

I

Immune system, boosting, 173, 182, 184
Implementation, 98–99
Implied consent, 59
Individualized approach, 92
Infertility, 136
Information, disclosure of
by clients, 175
by reflexologist, 58
Informed consent see Consent
Ingham, Eunice, 6, 18–19
Initial contact, 97–98
Injuries
reflexologist, 104
seven stages of injury, **105**
Institute for Complementary Medicine, 35
Insurance, professional indemnity, 18, 56, 143
Integrating reflexology, conventional
healthcare settings, 121–130
approaches to provision, 126–127, **128**
'busyness', acute hospital care, 123–124
complementary therapy committees, 123
differences, provision in hospital, 125–126
evidence for integrating, 124–125
management and supervisory issues, 127,
129
recommendations, 130
International Institute of Reflexology, 19
Interpersonal relations model, Peplau, 96
Interpersonal skills, 81
see also Communication
Intravenous cannula insertion site, 155

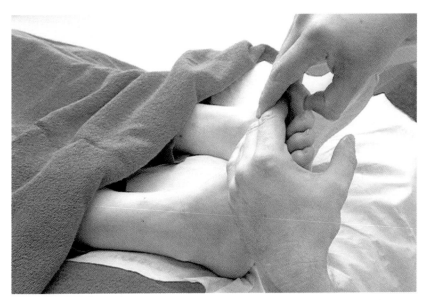

Plate 1   (Fig. 3.2, p. 40) Practitioner working the pituitary area. Photo courtesy of Katie Spruce BA (Hons), medical photographer, Christie Hospital NHS Trust, with permission.

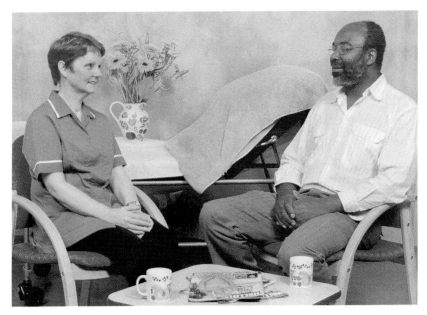

Plate 5   (Fig. 7.1, p. 94) Establishing the client–patient relationship. Permissions from subjects of photo is hereby ackknowledged.

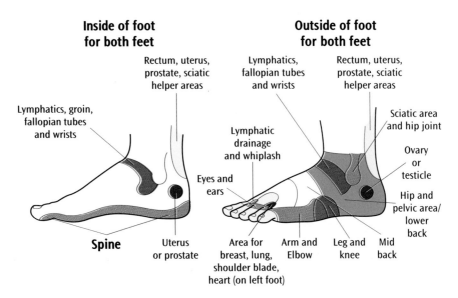

Inside of foot for both feet

Rectum, uterus, prostate, sciatic helper areas

Lymphatics, groin, fallopian tubes and wrists

Spine

Uterus or prostate

Outside of foot for both feet

Lymphatics, fallopian tubes and wrists

Rectum, uterus, prostate, sciatic helper areas

Lymphatic drainage and whiplash

Eyes and ears

Sciatic area and hip joint

Ovary or testicle

Hip and pelvic area/ lower back

Area for breast, lung, shoulder blade, heart (on left foot)

Arm and Elbow

Leg and knee

Mid back

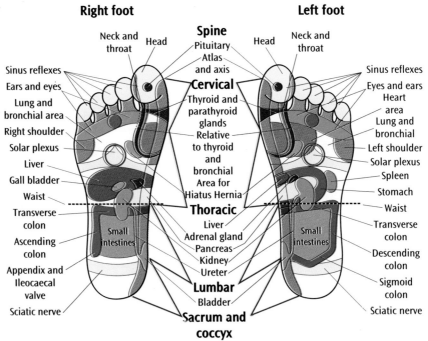

Right foot

Neck and throat

Head

Sinus reflexes

Ears and eyes

Lung and bronchial area

Right shoulder

Solar plexus

Liver

Gall bladder

Waist

Transverse colon

Ascending colon

Small intestines

Appendix and Ileocaecal valve

Sciatic nerve

Left foot

Head

Neck and throat

Sinus reflexes

Eyes and ears

Heart area

Lung and bronchial

Left shoulder

Solar plexus

Spleen

Stomach

Waist

Transverse colon

Small intestines

Descending colon

Sigmoid colon

Sciatic nerve

Spine

Pituitary

Atlas and axis

Cervical

Thyroid and parathyroid glands

Relative to thyroid and bronchial

Area for Hiatus Hernia

Thoracic

Liver

Adrenal gland

Pancreas

Kidney

Ureter

Lumbar

Bladder

Sacrum and coccyx

Plate 2   (Appendix, p. 49) Map 1: Reflexology foot chart (© Clive O'Hara 1981, 1991).

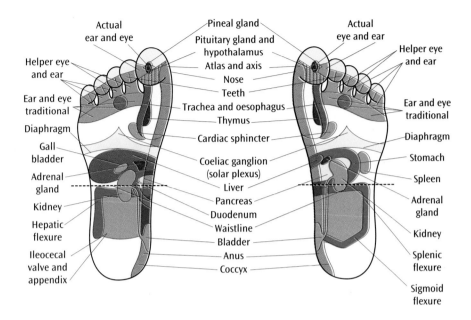

Actual ear and eye — Pineal gland — Actual eye and ear

Helper eye and ear — Pituitary gland and hypothalamus — Helper eye and ear

Ear and eye traditional — Atlas and axis — Nose — Teeth — Ear and eye traditional

Diaphragm — Trachea and oesophagus — Diaphragm

Gall bladder — Thymus — Stomach

Adrenal gland — Cardiac sphincter — Spleen

Kidney — Coeliac ganglion (solar plexus) — Adrenal gland

Hepatic flexure — Liver — Kidney

Ileocecal valve and appendix — Pancreas — Duodenum — Waistline — Bladder — Anus — Coccyx — Splenic flexure

Sigmoid flexure

Right foot   **Left foot**

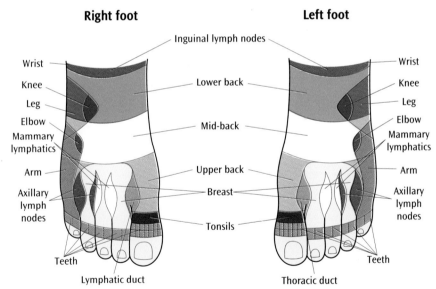

Inguinal lymph nodes

Wrist — Wrist

Knee — Lower back — Knee

Leg — Leg

Elbow — Mid-back — Elbow

Mammary lymphatics — Mammary lymphatics

Arm — Upper back — Arm

Axillary lymph nodes — Breast — Axillary lymph nodes

Tonsils

Teeth — Teeth

Lymphatic duct — Thoracic duct

Plate 3 (Appendix, p. 50) Map 2: Reflexology foot chart (© Clive O'Hara 1996).
Map 2 is intended as a supplement and does not include all the reflex areas from Map 1.

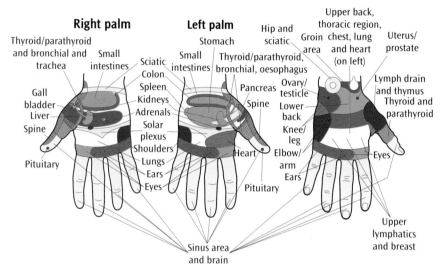

Back of hand (right and left)

Right palm

Thyroid/parathyroid and bronchial and trachea
Small intestines
Sciatic
Colon
Spleen
Kidneys
Adrenals
Solar plexus
Shoulders
Lungs
Ears
Eyes
Gall bladder
Liver
Spine
Pituitary

Left palm

Stomach
Small intestines
Thyroid/parathyroid, bronchial, oesophagus
Pancreas
Spine
Heart
Pituitary

Hip and sciatic
Groin area
Upper back, thoracic region, chest, lung and heart (on left)
Uterus/prostate
Ovary/testicle
Lower back
Knee/leg
Elbow/arm
Ears
Lymph drain and thymus
Thyroid and parathyroid
Eyes
Upper lymphatics and breast

Sinus area and brain

Plate 4   (Appendix, p. 51) Map 3: Reflexology hand chart (© Clive O'Hara 1991).

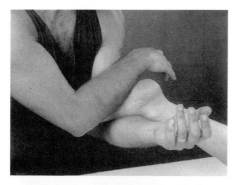

Plate 6 (Fig. 8.3, p. 112) The 'foot mangle' technique. The client is lying prone.

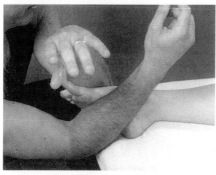

Plate 7 (Fig. 8.4, p. 112) The 'foot mangle' technique. The client is lying supine.

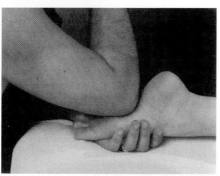

Plate 8 (Fig. 8.5, p. 113) The 'reflexor' technique. The client is lying prone.

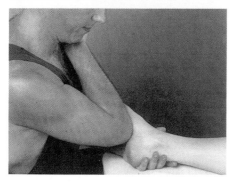

Plate 9 (Fig. 8.6, p. 114) The 'reflexor' technique. The client is lying supine.

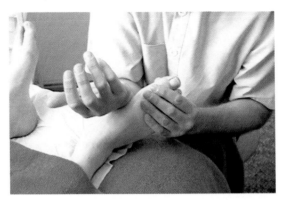

Plate 10 (Fig. 8.7, p. 114) Another illustration of using a surface of the forearm for reflexology. Photo courtesy of Katie Spruce BA (Hons), medical photographer, Christie Hospital NHS Trust, with permission.

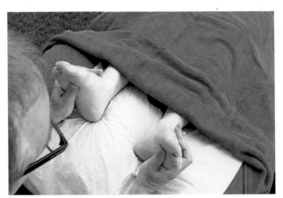

Plate 11 (Fig. 9.1, p. 124) Practitioner making contact with the feet. Photo courtesy of Katie Spruce BA (Hons), medical photographer, Christie Hospital NHS Trust, with permission.

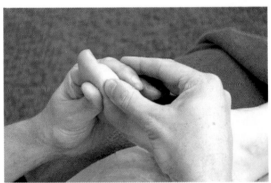

Plate 12 (Fig. 10.2, p. 142) Practitioner working the neck area. Photo courtesy of Katie Spruce BA (Hons), medical photographer, Christie Hospital NHS Trust, with permission.

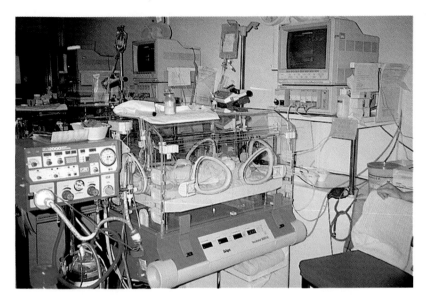

Plate 13   (Fig. 11.1, p. 149) General view of a neonatal unit.

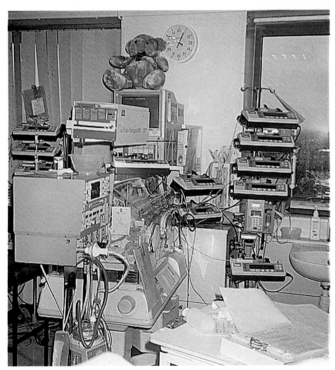

Plate 14   (Fig. 11.2, p. 151) Incubator and equipment.

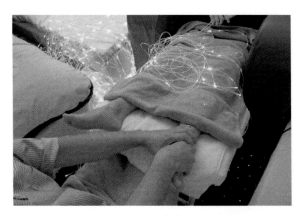

Plate 15 (Fig. 12.1, p. 163) Snoezelen therapy. Photo courtesy of Katie Spruce BA (Hons), medical photographer, Christie Hospital NHS Trust, with permission.

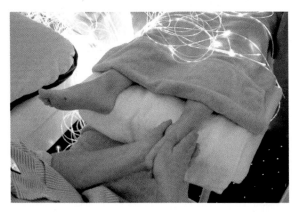

Plate 16 (Fig. 12.2, p. 164) Snoezelen therapy. Photo courtesy of Katie Spruce BA (Hons), medical photographer, Christie Hospital NHS Trust, with permission.

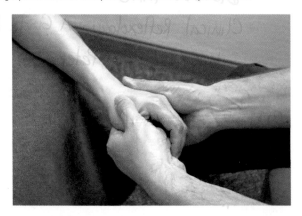

Plate 17 (Fig. 14.1. p. 188) Practitioner working at the bedside on the hand. Photo courtesy of Katie Spruce BA (Hons), medical photographer, Christie Hospital NHS Trust, with permission.